Preface

I have one mission in writing this book; it is to make women aware that they have more options than they thought possible when it comes to their abnormal periods. By knowing this one fact, that there are options, women don't have to be trapped into the world of synthetic pharmaceuticals-if they don't want to. I know firsthand that these pharmaceutical options can do more harm than good in some cases.

Nature often has everything people need to help their bodies have a normal period. This simple fact is life-changing if you know how to harness the power of what the earth gives us.

While I don't claim to be an expert in hormones, I also know that no one is truly an expert in women's hormones and our organs. How do I know this? Research related to women's health largely didn't start until 1993, when women's inclusion in research became law by the National Institutes of health[1]. That was a wee 30 years ago.

You may know that birth control was invented in the 1950s, but it was invented by men[2]. And as such, the testing on it was more for their benefit and not ours. For example, those women who were first tested on "the pill" who reported side effects were considered "unreliable participants." Many of these women were tested on without their informed consent, which is also a major human rights violation[2-3]. Some of them even died from these experiments. Today's birth control is a bit more refined than it was in the 1950s, but many women like me don't want the side effects that these hormones bring. They want a natural, healthy period that isn't masked by the pill.

On a related note, did you know that when you take the pill, you don't ovulate? How can that be the main solution to birth control and period health? While I truly support women who are on the pill because it provides freedom from pregnancy, it isn't tolerable for some and miserable to take for many.

Natural Medicine Silenced By Big Pharma

What I do claim to be an expert in is research, but you should know that research in natural medicine is systematically silenced by powerful forces, including Big Pharma. For more than three decades, during graduate school and afterward, I have immersed myself in the National Library of Medicine. Early on, I learned that preventive medicine and herbal research are rarely, if ever, disseminated to doctors. I have a deep desire to do better for myself and my patients. Because of this, I have uncovered research gems about natural medicine that can help people. And I'm here to help you. I've had help from my wonderful naturopath along the way, but a lot of what I know is by tirelessly looking for answers.

As a registered dietitian for more than 25 years, I know there is a better way for women's health. By studying herbs, natural medicines, and food-related strategies to overcome hormonal issues, I have much to share with the world. This comes full circle with my mission in writing this book: to share the vast array of options that get little mention in this world otherwise. And I know that you can, like me, learn not only to embrace being a woman but to enjoy the ebbs and flows that give us our strength.

These research gems I have discovered about natural healing aren't shared in medical schools because of a long-standing separation of natural medicine from medical schools. This separation was single-highhandedly established by the cunning actions of one man named Abraham Flexner who shut down any medical school if they were teaching natural medicines back in the early 1900s[4]. He was hired by the coffers of the Carnegie Foundation, with big influence from John D. Rockefeller and Andrew Carnegie. These capitalists also happened to be cashing in on pharmaceuticals made from chemicals derived from oil. They wielded their power by turning these oil chemicals into drugs. For these reasons the current medical system generally shuns natural medicines, whether there is research behind these natural medicines or not.

As you can imagine, there are a lot of greedy forces still alive and well that would lose a lot of money if people used natural medicine. For example, I suspect that Big Pharma and Big Food love to keep this message alive: "Herbs and supplements aren't regulated by the FDA." Yet the FDA's existence is largely based on Big Pharma. After all, a major task that they perform is to evaluate Big Pharma's research. Most people don't realize that the FDA isn't conducting research. They oversee research funded by the bottomless pocketbooks of Big Pharma. Many of the current gold-standard health recommendations also are influenced by Big Pharma as a result. And this is why it is so hard for any honest healthcare professional to find natural and practical solutions for health. You have to know what you are looking for to find it, and if Big Pharma and Big Food aren't distributing it, good luck finding the information. That is, unless you are a skeptic like I am and search tirelessly for the truth. *Up-to-Date* is a source for practitioners that is considered in high regard unless it comes to vitamins, minerals, and herbals, in which case it should be called *In-The-Dark*. Additionally, only 5% of National Institutes of Health resources are funneled to nutrition[5]. Perhaps it should be called the National Institute of Big Pharma instead.

My goal in life is to change how information is disseminated by being a voice for logic and careful observation combined with a true risk-benefit analysis of food, herbs, and supplements. This holistic risk-benefit analysis is completely lacking in all levels of conventional medical training at this point. In contrast, it is extensively discussed and used in the realm of functional medicine. Functional medicine is the advanced medical practice of getting to the root causes of health issues. Here are some examples of risk-benefit analysis that we use as functional medicine practitioners to evaluate an herb, nutrient, or supplement:

- What are the traditional uses?
- How are these uses supported in research?
- Are there any negative case reports of its use?
- What are the potential benefits?
- What are the potential risks?
- Does the duration of consumption make a difference in risk?
- Is there **synergism** with other **compounds**?
- Are there any interactions with medications or other compounds for the individual using it?
- Does the patient have a personal history of a positive or negative response to the compound?

By doing careful risk-benefit analysis of natural compounds over many decades, I've learned that most often, nature gets it right for us if we pay close attention. Our body heals when we give it what it needs. We as humans in Western society are never deficient in a drug, but often deficient in food, nutrients, and healing compounds.

In this book, I will dive into the pitfalls of current healthcare for women's menstrual cycles. I will dig deeply into the research and share with you discoveries that aren't discussed in most medical circles. At a minimum, I will give you ideas of how to empower yourself to ask the right questions when you go to the doctor, midwife, naturopath, or other healthcare provider of your choice. You deserve more choices.

1. History of Women's Participation in Clinical Research, Office of Research on Women's Health, NIH https://orwh.od.nih.gov/toolkit/recruitment/history
2. Blakemore, E., & Blakemore, E. (2023, August 24). *The first birth control pill used Puerto Rican women as guinea pigs.* HISTORY. https://www.history.com/news/birth-control-pill-history-puerto-rico-enovid
3. Liao PV, Dollin J. Half a century of the oral contraceptive pill: historical review and view to the future. Can Fam Physician. 2012 Dec;58(12):e757-60. PMID: 23242907; PMCID: PMC3520685. https://www.ncbi.nlm.nih.gov/pmc/articles/PMC3520685/
4. Stahnisch FW, Verhoef M. The flexner report of 1910 and its impact on complementary and alternative medicine and psychiatry in north america in the 20th century. Evid Based Complement Alternat Med. 2012;2012:647896. doi: 10.1155/2012/647896. Epub 2012 Dec 26. https://www.ncbi.nlm.nih.gov/pmc/articles/PMC3543812/
5. NIH Nutrition Report Executive Summary 2020-2021. https://dpcpsi.nih.gov/sites/default/files/NIH-Nutrition-Research-Report-Executive-Summary-508.pdf

Acknowledgments

I want to thank my daughter, Josie, for her thoughtful editing, her amazingly grounded personality, and sense of humor. Without her, this book wouldn't be possible. I also want to thank my own mother for her resilience and strength in raising 7 of her own children despite all the obstacles her own periods and reproductive issues caused her.

I

Part One

Part Two

One

Chapter 1

Periods Ruled My Life

Periods have dictated a lot of my life. This isn't all a bad thing. My periods have helped me to grow and learn as a health professional and as a woman. But almost every woman I know, in one way or another, has been plagued by emotional and physical aspects of their periods like me. These period issues are rampant, so I'm sure my story will resonate with you in one way or another. Most women I have ever known have similar stories that were either not addressed by their providers or were given only one solution: cover it all up with a synthetic pill.

The other side of the coin is that periods are empowering, power-ful, and life-giving when we choose to give our body what it needs. I believe that one of the greatest powers we have as women over men resides in our periods and the transformative changes we can have as a result of this cycle. And when we look at another positive angle, a healthy period can be exceptionally cathartic. By harnessing our uterine health, we can become omnipotent as intuitive and strong beings. After all, in both a physical and metaphorical sense, the uterus is the most powerful organ in the human body.

Heavy Pain and Heavy Flow

To say that periods ruled my life from day one is an understatement.

I was 13 years old, having my first period, without a clue, and doubled over in pain. And the bleeding was like a raging crimson river. Holy shit. No one told me the embarrassing number of tampons and pads I would bleed through month after month and year after year. I became weak, tired, and felt feeble being a woman as the years went by. The massive amount of blood loss and pain takes a toll on the body's strength and the brain's stamina. How can this be what we as women should endure? And the pain was unbearable. But I assumed every girl felt like this.

Back in the day, it was embarrassing to talk about tampon size and pad size and what it meant. I truly thought that needing a big tampon meant I was deformed or weird or abnormal or all of the above. No joke, this is what I thought at first. How wrong I was, but I had no point of reference and no one to discuss it with.

The force of gravity from the exceptionally muscular uterus pushes a lot of blood out at once, so of course you are going to bleed out of your tampon and pad. You need a large dam, or super plus tampon, to prevent the flow ma'am. And for me, even that wasn't enough. I stained a lot of my panties and ruined a lot of pants.

So what caused the flood? A demonish uterus or malnourished uterus? In my case and for countless women, the truth is that the uterus is malnourished and inflamed; we will deep dive this topic in this book.

Chapter 1

"What is wrong with me"? Too embarrassed to do anything, one of my sisters finally determined that all the abdominal pain issues that I had were coming from-my period. It took a while to learn this because she was already living on her own with kids of her own. But because my mom never got these horrible pains, she didn't know how to help or what was wrong.

When it came to the birds and bees talk I got as I hit my period, it consisted of my mother saying nothing, but to her credit, I was too scared to ask about it. I knew nothing about women's health other than the silly drawings of a woman's uterus and vagina and the wonderful revelation that you will get a period every 28-32 days back in gym class during 5th grade. Unfortunately, my mom was subjected to the shame around women's health just like all women were in the past. She endured period issues much like me and is a beacon of what it means to be strong at age 89 after having 7 children. Thankfully we can talk about these issues now and she is very happy I'm writing this book to help people. And I feel like that is all that matters now.

But looking back, there is so much I could have done if I would have only had the tools at the time. At 50 years old now, I sure wish that someone had shared with me the wisdom that I have had to learn the hard way over the years.

No one would go to the doctor for these things back in the day for the horror of discussing anything related to a woman's body. I took Tylenol, but it didn't touch the pain. Ibuprofen had just hit the shelves, but we didn't have any of that because it was new on the market.

A normal period? What do you mean? Aren't they all horrible like mine? As it turns out, no. My periods were not normal. As we know a "normal period" doesn't really exist. While a stigma still enfolds our menstrual cycles and cycle concerns, we can talk about it today. That is why I'm going to talk about it with frank honesty and show you how to achieve a more comfortable period using food and safe remedies.

A Heavy Period, Finally Defined

What is a heavy period, Dr. Google? More than ⅓ cup of blood loss throughout your menstrual cycle is technically a heavy period. I lost much more in a single hour before I started employing the strategies I show you in this book.

Eventually I did get some ibuprofen as a young teen, which helped the pain somewhat, but I had to reach for the bottle every 4 hours which ultimately caused my stomach to feel horrible every month. So my cyclic 25-day dread of my all-too-frequent and very heavy bleeding began. It was accompanied by severe pain and was a major issue in my life for the better part of 25 years. The ibuprofen didn't make a difference in the bleeding for me either.

Birth Control Mishaps

Like the ranks of most women, my doctor suggested I should try birth control to regulate my periods. I gave it a try. The first "pill" made me vomit but I was determined to stick it out. I did for a few months. Sure, my periods were more "normal," but nausea, vomiting, and a complete lack of emotions were my constant companions. I'm not kidding-the "pill" made all my emotions go away and affectionately in healthcare this is called anhedonia. It was a miserable time in my life and I never want to experience it again because I love life and the natural lows and highs that come with it emotionally.

I tried the Nuvaring® on the advice of another doctor because, supposedly, the hormones weren't able to reach the bloodstream in any significant way. It made me vomit more violently than the pill so I threw it away. So much for it not reaching my blood. How did this bit of garbage advice at the time pass muster?

Mid Cycle Ovary Pain-Oh Yay!

As I approached my late twenties, I began to be plagued with mid-cycle ovary pain each and every month. They called it Mittelschmerz, which essentially means mid-cycle ovary pain with no known cause. Super helpful, right? Granted, I got a break from it the two times I was pregnant, if you can call it that, because pregnancy was a whole other level of exhaustive challenges. But my body, clever as it was, was sure to give me Aunt Flo by 2 months after delivering my babies even though I was solely breastfeeding my babies. Lucky me!

Guess what my ovarian pain solution was? Take more ibuprofen for 14 days of the month or get on the pill. Sound like every other piece of advice? Yep! I'll skip the nausea, vomiting, and anhedonia due to the pill or the risk of kidney failure due to ibuprofen, thank you very much.

Instead, I fixed my ovarian pain myself by using natural medicine. After being fed up with my ovary pain, I went to a health food store. I grabbed a bottle of natural broccoli extracts and herbs called "Estrosense" which contains broccoli compounds, milk thistle, turmeric, and green tea extract. Within 1 month, my ovarian pain was gone. With broccoli and some herbs???? It was that simple. My doctor wanted me to take something that made me sick or put my kidneys in danger. I fixed it with broccoli and herbs. My period pain also got much better. While this exact supplement brand is a bit hard to find, there are similar products and I discuss these supplements throughout the book.

Turning to Natural Medicine for Good

Besides my ovarian pain recovery story, it took one monumental Halloween day to finally wake up and decide I needed to do something majorly different with my hormone health in terms of my heavy periods. My children and I were going trick-or-treating and my period had already started. Determined to have a good time, I made sure to put on a fresh maxi pad and super tampon before we left. Within 20 minutes I had already bled through my jeans. I had to go home in a hurry to change. Within the same hour, I filled yet another maxi pad and super tampon. This couldn't be good or normal.

After that day, I began researching nutrition and periods, and I found some surprising answers. I also started seeing a very wise naturopathic doctor, who has helped me tremendously.

I was 43 years old before learning what a normal period should be like and I work in healthcare. That is how little it is talked about. Maybe I wasn't asking the right questions, but "how often do you bleed through a tampon" should be one of the first questions a doctor should ask.

So at that point, I turned to the National Library of Medicine as well as Dr. Google. The secrecy and shame around periods haven't changed all that much over the years. And that is exactly why I'm writing this book-so that I can hopefully help you change the trajectory of your menstrual cycles or your daughters'. Or your Aunt or niece. Or any woman who is willing to look at our body's system differently than is explored in the short visits that you may have with your doctor's office.

As I entered the perimenopausal years, bleeding became erratic and sometimes severe. While this isn't uncommon for women, I wasn't going to rely on conventional medicine approaches only. After a "normal" physical exam and pap smear, I added even more natural approaches to my daily routine. These natural remedies helped me quickly and effectively achieve a gentle menstrual cycle again. I'm forever thankful for these and so I'll share with you how I did it throughout this book.

Things Haven't Changed for the Better

As I watch my daughter grow into an adult herself, I also watch almost every one of her friends start on birth control to regulate their periods. From a holistic perspective, this is entirely shocking and completely backward. I asked her friends if their doctors reviewed the nutritional components that make a healthy hormone pattern and a healthy uterus. They all looked at me uniformly with a puzzled look as if to say "what do you mean?" Not only is it not reviewed in depth at their doctors' visits, there is often zero discussion about diet and lifestyle when these young girls, or any woman at to the doctor's offices.

This is tragic. And I've been there. Even though we can talk more freely about women's health today, our current medical system doesn't have much of anything but synthetic hormones. I should know; I've seen many doctors over the years for the same issues and got the same answers: birth control and ibuprofen. And if you have these issues long enough, they may recommend a **hysterectomy** or an **endometrial ablation**. None of these treatments get to the root problem. None of them come without some serious risks. While diagnostics are useful and I wholeheartedly recommend you see your doctor for these, visits with the doctor rarely get to the root cause of your period issues.

Providers are caring and helpful. Many give their hearts and souls over to their practices. But they're taught what they're taught and this happens to be under the lens of a biased and greed-driven system. Their time often isn't their own and the current medical model shuns them for thinking and practicing outside the box. Every doctor or healthcare provider I've talked to admits that they are powerless to do differently based on the healthcare systems they work for. Every business and conglomerate strives to make more money with less time and less resources. How is a doctor to fight against this system effectively? They usually can't unless they put their necks out and risk their income and credibility forced upon them by the so-called gold standards; pharmaceuticals.

Miseducation in Healthcare

I also didn't learn how nutrients affect hormones in my graduate nutritional sciences program; therefore I can't be too harsh on the current physician medical system. Everything I know today was either self-taught or learned from my functional medicine training, my research, and my naturopathic doctor. That's not to say I didn't learn a lot in school. I just didn't learn what I needed to learn.

When it comes to hormonal health, there are still a lot of unknowns in terms of scientific evidence. You should not let this stop you from trying to get well. If you are hesitant and resort to conventional medicine, you may suffer for 25 years (or more) like I did. Because you picked up this book, I bet you also are trying to think outside of the box and find natural ways to heal your reproductive organs.

For thousands of years, women used herbal medicine and natural medicine to help balance hormonal issues. The advent of modern medicine took that all away from us for the exact reason you might think: money and greed of powerful people like Flexner.[1] All so that money would only be funneled in the direction of pharmaceuticals because of their push to make drugs to fatten more rich people's pocketbooks.

It makes me mad. I've had undue suffering which could have been prevented if my doctors had been trained in herbal medicine and nutritional healing.

Chapter 1

It's not their fault they are trained what they are trained, but it is fully lacking any traditional medicines. And their pharmaceutical tools are very limited at best for women's health. Big Pharma keeps it that way by continuing to keep the machine moving in the same direction and forcing the doubts you have about using what the earth has given us.

What tools do the current average physicians get for abnormal period pain and bleeding? Take ibuprofen or take birth control. I'm not joking; this is really it for the most part. If you have **endometriosis** or polycystic ovarian syndrome, you are given very dire options -synthetic hormones or going under the knife.

Despite my lifelong period issues, diagnostics were only offered once: when I had an ovarian cyst burst. Not after a lifetime of abnormal periods. I didn't get the diagnostics I needed or deserved. Ever. Get your pap smear and be on your way, ma'am. Pap smears are critical and life-saving so you should do them. They just aren't enough if you are suffering from most women's issues. Your pap smear didn't show anything? Well, good luck and have fun with abnormal periods, according to the current medical model.

That wasn't good enough for me. I knew there had to be answers in nature because nature is smart that way. Luckily for me, I did receive an undergraduate degree in nutrition and a master's degree in nutritional science where I learned I could always dive deeply into the sea of clinical research. I also have conducted multiple clinical research projects, so I was no stranger to interpreting the science.

In this book, I'll walk you through what has worked for me from a nutritional standpoint, the research that we have today about nutritional factors for period and hormonal health, and the natural time-honored and clinically proven herbal remedies that are safe to try once you are cleared to do so by your healthcare provider.

What This Book Is

This book is a review of natural solutions for period issues. We delve into how nutrients and herbs work to support your hormonal balance. After all, you can't have healthy organs and hormones without nourishing them.

What This Book Isn't

While there are a lot of safe things to try in this book after you discuss them with your healthcare provider, it isn't a replacement for seeking out routine care and follow-ups with your provider when needed. You should always see your provider if you have any symptoms that are out of the range of normal. Please do get your routine PAP smears and follow-ups.

Chapter 1 References

1. Stahnisch FW, Verhoef M. The flexner report of 1910 and its impact on complementary and alternative medicine and psychiatry in north america in the 20th century. Evid Based Complement Alternat Med. 2012;2012:647896. doi: 10.1155/2012/647896. Epub 2012 Dec 26. https://www.ncbi.nlm.nih.gov/pmc/articles/PMC3543812/

Chapter 2

All About Periods and Hormones

> "A pure heart and mind only takes you so far - sooner or later the hormones have their say, too."
> **-Jim Butcher**

In this chapter, I break down the essential understanding of hormones and how they affect you. By doing so, you can understand how natural approaches can help balance your hormones to create a healthier period and healthier uterus.

Normal is a Novelty

It's kind of laughable if you try to research what a normal period is and what is abnormal. Periods can come every 21-35 days and you can bleed from 2-7 days according to the Mayo Clinic.[1]

The clinic website goes on to say that you should seek medical care if you have heavy bleeding (soaking through a tampon or pad every hour or two), bleeding for longer than 7 days, severe pain, bleeding between periods, and many other criteria such as infrequent bleeding, fevers, etc. A normal period ideally would also be free of premenstrual syndrome symptoms and pain.

Based on this criteria, I would have had to go to the doctor every month of my life until I found nutritional and herbal solutions to help myself.

From this description, I don't know many women who have the pleasure of having a normal menstrual cycle. My suspicion for the reason that so many women struggle to have a normal period is because of our poor food supply, lack of time-honored herbs, and lack of nutrients. It is also because we are told to follow the US Dietary Guidelines, which would ultimately leave most women lacking in the proper amount of nutrients they need for a healthy period.

This suspicion is based on personal experience and from other women I've known who change their diet and lifestyle and their periods improve. It is also based on the research that shows how much nutrients are needed to properly make hormones and to support a strong and healthy uterus.

No offense to the vegan movement but as a whole would leave some women like me in dire hormonal health because of the lack of hormonal precursors needed for a normal cycle. I will describe the issues with this type of diet for periods as we go along.

Chapter 2

The Ping Pong Game of Hormones

Hormones are similar to a game of ping pong. With the right finesse, the game of hormones goes on well. However, the ball of hormones easily flies off the table if all conditions aren't perfect. That's why I compare hormones to a ping-pong game.

If you want to have a manageable period you have to understand that balanced hormones are central to this. Hormones aren't the only factor in having a healthy period, they are a major factor. By having some basic knowledge of these hormones and what they do, you can be on your way to a better monthly flow.

Here I will review the following hormones and their effects on your periods:

- Cortisol
- Thyroid Hormone
- Insulin
- Estrogen
- Progesterone
- Testosterone
- Calcitriol
- DHEA

To say that hormones are complicated is putting it mildly. All hormones interact with other hormones. You may be eating the proper nutrients to support insulin, but completely wrecking what is needed to make normal thyroid hormones. Balance and nuance are needed. But it's a ping-pong game, meaning hormones all bounce off of each other and if one gets thrown off, the game is over for periods being normal.

Don't despair; I'll show you how you can support all hormones.

I'm not going to discuss every hormone in the human body, but will discuss those that you can safely and positively change with simple diet and lifestyle changes.

* * *

How About Hormone Testing?

> Hormones not only fluctuate throughout your menstrual cycle, they fluctuate during each day. Cortisol, the hormone that controls inflammation and the stress response, naturally peaks in the morning and subsides as the day goes on. But, if your cortisol is elevated all day long, your other hormones will be blunted. The DUTCH test is a reliable way of testing your hormone fluctuations throughout the day by measuring hormones in your urine.
>
> The DUTCH test is an analysis of 35 different hormones, including DHEA, estrogen, progesterone, melatonin, testosterone, and cortisol. It measures neurotransmitters including dopamine and norepinephrine. As a bonus, it checks vitamin **metabolites** that may help identify core nutritional imbalances that are causing some of your hormone levels to be off.
>
> While conventional doctors often don't use this test, the reasoning behind not using it remains elusive. The DUTCH test really helps women become more aware of their hormone issues.
>
> Research shows the DUTCH test is a reliable test for measuring such hormones. Most conventional doctors will order one-time progesterone, estrogen, and testosterone, but this doesn't tell the whole story as you read about in the cortisol section.[2-4]

Chapter 2

The DUTCH test has improved my life by allowing me to identify the core hormone issues that were driving my perimenopausal symptoms. By addressing these core issues, I have more energy, focus, and vitality. These core issues will be described throughout this book.

* * *

Backhanded Cortisol

The first hormone I will describe is cortisol. It is the stress hormone that will make or break all hormones in the body. Not all cortisol is bad because healthy levels of cortisol help the body be alert, focused, and even dampens **inflammation** while regulating blood pressure. But, too much cortisol causes almost all other hormones to be lower than they should be. This is affectionately called the "**cortisol steal**". If you have too much stress which drives up cortisol, you can't have normal hormones including testosterone.[5] And your thyroid hormone and insulin won't be normal either. It is paramount you manage your hormones by managing the stress in your life to ultimately help normalize hormones.

As many health experts are learning, much of our stress begins in the gut, which is why the gut-brain axis is critical. In other words, by nourishing and healing your gut, you can make a lot of headway into managing your stress and cortisol levels. In my book Gut Fix, I describe in great depth ways that you can heal your gut which ultimately helps dampen stress. But ultimately, if you have a high-stress lifestyle, you will seriously need to figure out your health priorities and what you are willing to accept. You won't have a normal period if you can't manage your stress due to the cortisol steal.

If you want to learn more about the complexities of the cortisol response and how it reduces healthy hormone levels, you can visit Genova Diagnostics website.[6]

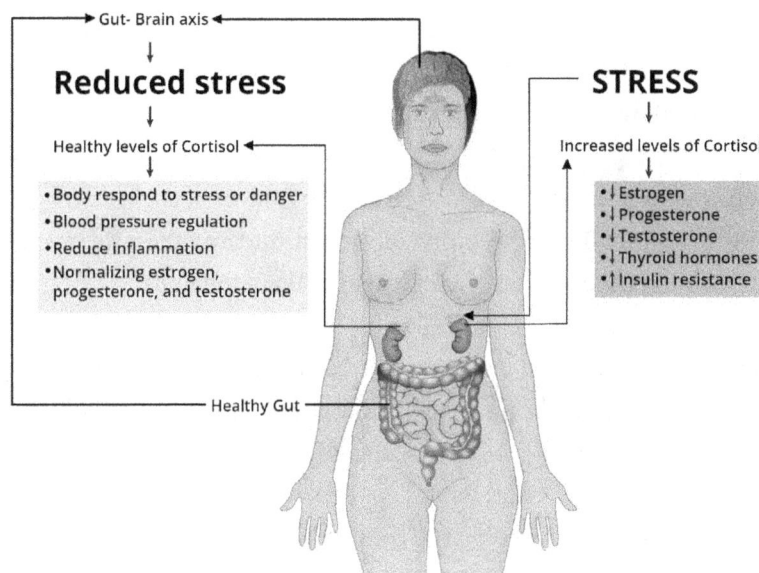

Figure 1: A graphic description of how cortisol robs the body of all sex hormones and drives thyroid and insulin imbalances. This image also describes how gut health counteracts the imbalances of stress and cortisol.

Thyroid Hormone-The Master Regulator

Sadly, many women in their lives will experience a thyroid problem at one point, including myself. Many health experts now understand that this is often related to dietary issues, nutrient deficiencies, and food sensitivities. A lot of people with thyroid imbalances have gluten **antibodies** and following a gluten-free diet can decrease thyroid antibodies[7]. This means that gluten is wreaking havoc with normal thyroid function for many. An imbalanced diet and **processed foods** are also a disaster for thyroid function.

To make things even more challenging, many common medications interfere with proper thyroid function, including antacids, beta blockers (blood pressure medication), seizure medication, birth control- yes you heard that right- and estrogen replacement.[8]

Ultimately, improper thyroid function affects your periods. This is because thyroid hormone, T_3 (Triiodothyronine), stimulates the release of the hormone called progesterone from **luteal cells** in the body.[9]

Both low and high thyroid levels are also related to having abnormal levels of estrogen and testosterone levels because thyroid hormone helps make estrogen and testosterone more available for the body to use.[10]

Thyroid is complicated so if you want to understand this topic more deeply, you can visit Thyroid Nutrition Educators.[11] Basically, lack of any nutrient can make your thyroid function abnormal, but the most well-studied nutrients that impact thyroid are vitamin D, iodine, B-vitamins, iron, selenium, protein, zinc, and selenium.

Insulin: The Backspin

Insulin is the hormone that helps cells receive sugar so that blood sugar levels don't become dangerously high. But most Americans these days are **insulin resistant**, so their bodies compensate by making a lot more insulin.

Too much insulin caused by this resistance causes women to make too much testosterone at the expense of estrogen. In fact, high insulin levels create estrogen deficiency.[12] For this reason, I consider insulin to be a backspin hormone.

High insulin levels increase growth hormone levels, which isn't a good thing when it comes to long-term health. Growth hormones trigger growth, and this can even make abnormal and dysfunctional cells multiply too. This is perhaps why people with insulin resistance have an increased risk of cancer and heart disease too. On the other hand, excess progesterone, another primarily women's hormone, can cause insulin resistance.[13]

For women with polycystic ovarian syndrome, insulin resistance is one of the major causes of the condition, so the goal in this case is to reduce insulin resistance as we will get into in Chapter 6. Too much insulin causes period issues, so a cornerstone to healthy periods is ditching a lot of junky carbohydrates in the diet and improving insulin levels. You can do so by eating nutrient-rich foods and taking key supplements that we will discuss throughout the book.

Estrogen: The Driver

Estrogen is the most well-known women's hormone because it makes women have certain characteristics, such as breasts and curvy hips. Importantly, estrogen is key for fertility and much more as well so that is why I coin it the driver here.[14]

But, this driver is very easily thrown off balance. As reviewed above, other hormones can cause estrogen to be too low, such as too much insulin, cortisol, or abnormal thyroid levels. So balancing those is critical to having an ideal amount of estrogen in your body over the years.

An important thing to know about estrogen is that there is more than one type of it. Some types of estrogen are more damaging to the body while others are generally beneficial.

There are two main types of estrogen that are good to be familiar with:

- Estriol (E3) is thought to be protective from diseases
- Estrone (E1) is implicated in diseases like cancer

In this book you will learn how to increase beneficial estrogen (E3) while decreasing harmful estrogen (E1) through food strategies and natural supplements.

Progesterone: The Counter Driver

Progesterone is another hormone that helps with fertility, but also helps prepare the uterus for pregnancy by causing a thickening of the uterus mid cycle. It also supports healthy pregnancy as well. Progesterone helps keep estrogen in check which is why I call it the counter driver.

Progesterone is also important for bone health and nerve health.[15]

Stress and imbalanced diet as well as nutrient deficiencies can cause both high and low progesterone levels by driving up cortisol levels. Too low of cholesterol levels can also cause a reduction in progesterone in the body. This means that a vegan diet can cause your progesterone levels to be too low. In fact, vegan diets generally may have negative effects on pregnancy outcomes and this could be related to its effects on hormones like progesterone.[16-17]

Problems with imbalances in progesterone affect fertility. Also, low progesterone levels can cause heavy periods, which no one wants. This is because low progesterone forces the body to become **estrogen dominant** and causes too much bleeding. The foods, nutrients, and herbs in this book help support natural progesterone balance.

All told, low progesterone plagues more women than too high of progesterone levels which leaves women estrogen dominant. This puts us at risk of all sorts of period problems and this book will help guide the normalization of progesterone in a natural way[17].

Testosterone: The Hidden Hormone in Women

While testosterone is generally thought of as a masculine hormone, women need it too. We need it to keep our energy levels normal and our moods balanced. It promotes bone health as well as muscle strength. Not only that, testosterone keeps women's interest in sex and ability to orgasm at normal levels.

Like the other hormones listed here, cortisol or stress can deplete testosterone levels and women with low levels can suffer from low mood and low sexual function.

However, too much testosterone decreases estrogen levels in the body. High testosterone is more common in women who have **polycystic ovarian syndrome**. This is also related to too much insulin in the body.[19]

While high testosterone levels are conventionally treated with medications such as **metformin**, spironolactone, and hormone therapy, there are natural approaches that can support healthy testosterone levels. And that's the whole point of this book. You will learn ways to naturally balance testosterone including meal timing, healthy fats, and healthy supplements.

Chapter 2

Calcitriol: The Sunny Game Saver

Calcitriol is a hormone that many don't know about, but most are familiar with its building block: vitamin D. As the only hormone that is made indirectly from the sunlight, calcitriol is in partial control of every hormone too. Vitamin D as calcitriol controls estrogen production in the body to some extent.[20]

Low vitamin D levels contribute to insulin resistance and abnormal thyroid function, which both then cause abnormal estrogen levels.[21] Optimal vitamin D levels are related to improved fertility and also help balance both estrogen and progesterone. Because of this, vitamin D is thought to help reduce the risk of breast cancer as well.[22-2]

Most people these days don't get enough vitamin D from the sun and also don't get enough from food, supplemental vitamin D is an important baseline nutrient for many people to help maintain normal hormone levels. I'll talk more about recommended doses in Chapter 4.

Your Inner Seasons

There is a lot of talk these days about women's seasons, which are the natural ebb and flow of hormones throughout your menstrual cycle. These fluctuations are a complicated symphony and I find that beyond understanding the basics of them, they only serve to be confusing for the average person. As such, I will explain the major shifts in your period seasons so that you can understand what all the talk is about on social media and what the trendy seed cycling means.

Your so-called normal 28-day cycle has 4 seasons when you are in the prime reproductive phase of your life. But you can throw these concepts out the window as you are in perimenopause and approaching menopause or have conditions like PCOS.

- **Winter**-this is when you are menstruating
- **Spring**-this is when estrogen begins to peak after your period is over
- **Summer**-estrogen is still peaking and you are ovulating and most fertile
- **Fall**-progesterone peaks and this is where your uterus is readying for pregnancy or for your next "winter" period

The natural ebb and flow of hormones are compared to seasons and are helpful because during Fall, you should slow down and take care and nurture your body because you are headed into the energy-intensive period, or "Winter" you are about to have. Lightly exercise but don't go all in on your physical activity during the fall. The same goes for Winter, only you may want to slow down even more so that your body's period losses don't put extra stress on your mental and physical health. Then, as Spring comes on you can ramp up your exercise a bit and do your peak physical activity during Summer.

Seed cycling is all over social media. This is essentially a recommendation to have certain foods that are seeds during different phases of your cycle, like having ground flax seeds and pumpkin seeds during Winter and Fall and then having sunflower seeds and sesame seeds during summer and fall. They say if you don't have a normal cycle, just cycle your seed intake according to the moon.

While these seeds might work for you, for me and many women I know, flaxseeds or other seeds can cause some of the most horrific gut pain likely related to their anti-nutrient content including **phytates**. All I'm saying is that if this is you, don't eat them. It's not worth the gut pain and there is no scientific validation for seed cycling in the first place. That said, if you like these seeds and find them beneficial without gut pain, go ahead and try seed cycling.

Flax seeds and sesame seeds on their own have a small amount of evidence that they may support hormone health. For example, flax seeds may help promote cycle regularity.[24] Sesame seeds may increase sex hormone binding globulin levels.[25] This hormone helps regulate the amount of other hormones that affect your body's tissues.

***

DHEA: Friend to Your Body?

DHEA is a prohormone and the parent of estrogen, progesterone, cortisol, DHEAS, and testosterone. As the parent hormone, DHEA has limitless possible benefits for many women. In fact, supplements of DHEA may improve fertility rates in women with endometriosis.[26] Further, low DHEA and testosterone levels are related to increased levels of period pain.[27] Eating healthy fat in the diet can help increase DHEA levels, but I highly recommend that you get your DHEA levels checked by your provider using the DUTCH hormone test. If you are like me, it can be very life-changing to test and treat DHEA appropriately. You may get your sex life back and you may feel normal again after using DHEA, like I did. In other words, don't fall prey to replacement of progesterone and estrogen without addressing DHEA as you get closer to menopause or if you have period problems! Monitor your DHEA levels and have your provider treat DHEA deficiency if you are low. While eating healthy foods can help support normal DHEA levels, our toxic environments may make it impossible to achieve normal DHEA levels on their own. I review more of the fascinating benefits of DHEA on page 187.

In summary, optimizing hormones requires a nuanced balance of foods, nutrients, and healing compounds that are the building blocks of every cell in our bodies. Learn more about how to optimize your hormones and your uterus for the best periods possible in Chapter 3-5.

Chapter 2 References

1. Menstrual Cycle: What's Normal, What's Not, Mayo Clinic. https://www.mayoclinic.org/healthy-lifestyle/womens-health/in-depth/menstrual-cycle/art-20047186#
2. Newman M, Curran DA. Reliability of a dried urine test for comprehensive assessment of urine hormones and metabolites. BMC Chem. 2021 Mar 15;15(1). https://pubmed.ncbi.nlm.nih.gov/33722278/
3. Wasalathanthri S, Tennekoon KH, Sufi S. Feasibility of using paper impregnated with urine instead of liquid urine for assessing ovarian activity. Ceylon Med J. 2003 Mar;48(1):4-6. https://pubmed.ncbi.nlm.nih.gov/12795010/
4. Study Supporting DUTCH Testing: Improved Serum Correlation. Mark Newman MS. https://dutchtest.com/blog/a-new-study-supporting-dutch-testing/
5. Whirledge S, Cidlowski JA. Glucocorticoids, stress, and fertility. Minerva Endocrinol. 2010 Jun;35(2):109-25. https://www.ncbi.nlm.nih.gov/pmc/articles/PMC3547681/
6. The Steroidogenic Pathway: Understanding What Influences Each Step, Genova Diagnostics 2016. https://www.gdx.net/files/clinicians/medical-education/previous-webinars/June-2016-The-Steroidogenic-Pathway-Understanding-What-Influences-Each-Step-Antoine.pdf
7. Krysiak R, Szkróbka W, Okopień B. The Effect of Gluten-Free Diet on Thyroid Autoimmunity in Drug-Naïve Women with Hashimoto's Thyroiditis: A Pilot Study. Exp Clin Endocrinol Diabetes. 2019 Jul;127(7):417-422. https://pubmed.ncbi.nlm.nih.gov/30060266/

8. Thyroid Function Test, American Thyroid Association https://www.thyroid.org/thyroid-function-tests/
9. Datta M, Roy P, Banerjee J, Bhattacharya S. Thyroid hormone stimulates progesterone release from human luteal cells by generating a proteinaceous factor. J Endocrinol. 1998 Sep;158(3):319-25. https://pubmed.ncbi.nlm.nih.gov/9846161/#
10. Kjaergaard AD, Marouli E, Papadopoulou A, Deloukas P, Kuś A, Sterenborg R, Teumer A, Burgess S, Åsvold BO, Chasman DI, Medici M, Ellervik C. Thyroid function, sex hormones and sexual function: a Mendelian randomization study. Eur J Epidemiol. 2021 Mar;36(3):335-344. https://www.ncbi.nlm.nih.gov/pmc/articles/PMC7612952/#
11. 5 Tests to Measure Optimum Thyroid Levels, Thyroid Nutrition Educators. https://www.thyroidnutritioneducators.com/5-tests-to-measure-optimum-thyroid-levels/
12. Suba Z. Interplay between insulin resistance and estrogen deficiency as co- activators in carcinogenesis. Pathol Oncol Res. 2012 Apr;18(2):123-33. https://pubmed.ncbi.nlm.nih.gov/21984197/#
13. Wada T, Hori S, Sugiyama M, Fujisawa E, Nakano T, Tsuneki H, Nagira K, Saito S, Sasaoka T. Progesterone inhibits glucose uptake by affecting diverse steps of insulin signaling in 3T3-L1 adipocytes. Am J Physiol Endocrinol Metab. 2010 Apr;298(4). https://pubmed.ncbi.nlm.nih.gov/20071559/
14. Hamilton KJ, Hewitt SC, Arao Y, Korach KS. Estrogen Hormone Biology. Curr Top Dev Biol. 2017;125:109-146. https://pubmed.ncbi.nlm.nih.gov/28527569/
15. Cable JK, Grider MH. Physiology, Progesterone. [Updated 2023 May 1]. In: StatPearls [Internet]. Treasure Island (FL): StatPearls Publishing; 2024 Jan-. https://www.ncbi.nlm.nih.gov/books/NBK558960/
16. Pirke KM, Schweiger U, Laessle R, Dickhaut B, Schweiger M, Waechtler M. Dieting influences the menstrual cycle: vegetarian versus nonvegetarian diet. Fertil Steril. 1986 Dec;46(6):1083-8. https://pubmed.ncbi.nlm.nih.gov/3096794/

17. Sebastiani G, Herranz Barbero A, Borrás-Novell C, Alsina Casanova M, Aldecoa-Bilbao V, Andreu-Fernández V, Pascual Tutusaus M, Ferrero Martínez S, Gómez Roig MD, García-Algar O. The Effects of Vegetarian and Vegan Diet during Pregnancy on the Health of Mothers and Offspring. Nutrients. 2019 Mar 6;11(3): 557. https://pubmed.ncbi.nlm.nih.gov/30845641/
18. Jewson M, Purohit P, Lumsden MA. Progesterone and abnormal uterine bleeding/menstrual disorders. Best Pract Res Clin Obstet Gynaecol. 2020 Nov;69:62-73. https://pubmed.ncbi.nlm.nih.gov/32698992/#
19. What Causes High Testosterone In Women? Medical News Today. https://www.medicalnewstoday.com/articles/321292#treatment
20. Kinuta K, Tanaka H, Moriwake T, Aya K, Kato S, Seino Y. Vitamin D is an important factor in estrogen biosynthesis of both women's and male gonads. Endocrinology. 2000 Apr;141(4):1317-24. https://pubmed.ncbi.nlm.nih.gov/10746634/
21. Chu C, Tsuprykov O, Chen X, Elitok S, Krämer BK, Hocher B. Relationship Between Vitamin D and Hormones Important for Human Fertility in Reproductive-Aged Women. Front Endocrinol (Lausanne). 2021 Apr 14;12:666687. https://www.ncbi.nlm.nih.gov/pmc/articles/PMC8081388/
22. Harmon QE, Kissell K, Jukic AMZ, Kim K, Sjaarda L, Perkins NJ, Umbach DM, Schisterman EF, Baird DD, Mumford SL. Vitamin D and Reproductive Hormones Across the Menstrual Cycle. Hum Reprod. 2020 Feb 29;35(2):413-423. https://pubmed.ncbi.nlm.nih.gov/32068843
23. Knight JA, Wong J, Blackmore KM, Raboud JM, Vieth R. Vitamin D association with estradiol and progesterone in young women. Cancer Causes Control. 2010 Mar;21(3):479-83. https://pubmed.ncbi.nlm.nih.gov/19916051/
24. Phipps WR, Martini MC, Lampe JW, Slavin JL, Kurzer MS. Effect of flax seed ingestion on the menstrual cycle. J Clin Endocrinol Metab. 1993 Nov;77(5):1215-9. https://www.ncbi.nlm.nih.gov/pubmed/8077314

25. Phipps WR, Martini MC, Lampe JW, Slavin JL, Kurzer MS. Effect of flax seed ingestion on the menstrual cycle. J Clin Endocrinol Metab. 1993 Nov;77(5):1215-9. https://www.ncbi.nlm.nih.gov/pubmed/8077314
26. Çelik Ö, Acet M, İmren A, Çelik N, Erşahin A, Aktun LH, Otlu B, Çelik S, Çalışkan E, Ünlü C. DHEA supplementation improves endometrial HOXA-10 mRNA expression in poor responders. J Turk Ger Gynecol Assoc. 2017 Dec 15;18(4):160-166. https://www.ncbi.nlm.nih.gov/pmc/articles/PMC5776153/
27. Evans SF, Kwok Y, Solterbeck A, Pyragius C, Hull ML, Hutchinson MR, Rolan P. The Relationship Between Androgens and Days per Month of Period Pain, Pelvic Pain, Headache, and TLR4 Responsiveness of Peripheral Blood Mononuclear Cells in Young Women with Dysmenorrhoea. J Pain Res. 2021 Mar 3;14:585-599. https://www.ncbi.nlm.nih.gov/pmc/articles/PMC7937378/

Three

Chapter 3

How to Build a Healthy Uterus With Food

Nutrients are the building blocks of absolutely everything in the body, so having a healthy period not only depends on healthy hormones as described above, but also on providing enough nutrients so the structure of the uterus and hormones are healthy too.

In this chapter, learn how foods play a critical role in helping prevent period issues. Also, learn about the food sources of where these nutrients come from and when supplementation of these nutrients can be helpful or harmful. We will dive more into dietary supplements and herbs in the upcoming chapters too.

Healing Foods-The Answer to Many Period Problems

You can't be healthy if you are low in nutrients-plain and simple. Eating a diet that is based on nutrient-dense foods should be the cornerstone of your healing hormonal journey. This is because women who eat a lot of processed foods have more period issues than those who don't.[1]

But, as you will learn throughout this chapter, it can be almost impossible to get enough nutrients in your diet alone if you have period problems. To help guide you through when and where to supplement, I will give you tips on confidently buying quality supplements in the next chapter.

Throughout the following chapters, I will give you suggestions of how to best get nutrients first from foods and how to get the nutrients from supplements when it becomes impossible to get enough from your diet. I will give you doses and forms of supplements to find so that you can get the best quality supplements on the market.

Cholesterol: The Backbone of ALL Hormones

Cholesterol gets a bad name, but nothing in the way of cholesterol is straightforward. When it comes to hormones, cholesterol is essential because it is the backbone of all **steroid hormones**. Every hormone we talked about in Chapter 1 depends on cholesterol because it makes up the structure of these hormones.

While the topic of cholesterol is controversial, some research points to the fact that cholesterol-lowering medications cause a decrease in hormone production and this isn't a good thing.[2]

Even more disturbing is that hormone studies using cholesterol medicines primarily study men and not women. But even men can have a reduction in hormones related to high-dose cholesterol medications[3]. However, for every study you see that cholesterol medicines interfere with hormones, there is another study that says they don't, so you should take this all with a grain of salt and carefully discuss your individual needs with your healthcare provider.

Some research shows that cholesterol medications significantly decrease hormone precursors in women, so careful consideration should be made for women taking statin cholesterol medications[4]. Additionally, dietary cholesterol isn't related to heart disease risk according to a review study in Nutrients journal[5].

However, if you have genetic risk factors for heart disease, such as the **ApoE4 genotype**, you may need to still be careful of foods that drive up cholesterol, such as saturated fat, even if you have hormonal imbalances.

Cholesterol from the diet comes from animal foods only. But, cholesterol is naturally made in the liver too. If you have been told that your cholesterol levels are too low, you may want to consider changing your diet to regularly contain foods that support healthy cholesterol levels, such as eggs, organ meats, wild-caught fatty fish, wild game, grass fed beef, poultry, and shellfish. In fact, these foods that have a lot of cholesterol are rich in other nutrients needed for a healthy uterus and hormones as we will discuss next.

Organ Meats-Superfoods for the Uterus

If you have heavy periods or irregular periods there is one food that I would recommend over all others: grass fed beef liver or chicken liver. Other organ meats are helpful too, and it's also a good idea to eat them as you can or take a grass fed organ meats supplement. You should eat liver because it has almost all of the nutrients you need to support healthy periods.

While not a popular food, it is the most nutritious food on the planet by far. It contains 13 mg of iron for just 4 ounces of beef liver. Liver contains ALL the vitamins and 9 vitamins with over ⅓ of your daily needs. There truly are no other foods that can compare for helping nourish your organs.

People worry about eating liver because it is the body's **toxin** filter. True.

Chapter 3

The good news, though, is that the liver doesn't store these toxins which means that when you eat liver, you aren't eating toxins. Rather, the liver cleans the body of toxins, along with the intestines and more, making them non-toxic. If you are wondering where toxins are stored, they are in the fat tissue of animals, not the liver. Examples of where it is stored include breast tissue, belly fat, and the brain. Liver has enzymes that clear out these toxins or neutralize them. Filters in the liver are enzymes, which may have some potent health benefits for you when you eat them. In contrast, a steak doesn't have these enzymes.

Yes, liver can taste great. There are many cooking techniques that make it more delicious than a rib steak. You can saute and grill liver. Marinate it in flavorful spices, especially garlic. Liver is fantastic as pate. For making liver fit easily into your diet, you can mix ground liver into meatballs, meat sauces, meatloaf, stuffing, soups, and just about any dish. You probably won't even notice it is there. If you want to know how to make liver taste good, visit Weston's Price's fascinating information about the liver.[6] You can find some tasty liver recipes in the recipe section of this book as well.

As much as I can extol the health benefits of liver as a super food, it may never fit your taste palate. If this is you, there are liver supplements out there for you. You can find countless brands of liver capsules on the market. Some are desiccated (fat removed), and some are not. Desiccation can mean that some nutrients are taken out too and some chemicals can be used in the desiccation process. It's best to do your research here. Find liver capsules from grass-fed, chemical-free animals, non-defatted, just as you would want to do if you are eating it. I like and use the ones from MK Supplements, Ancestral Supplements, Heart and Soil, and Dr. Kilz.

If you still can't see yourself doing this, the next best thing is eating fish roe, which is highly nutritious and has been revered since humans have existed for its benefits for hormonal health. It's kind of hard to come by, but I enjoy Tobiko fish eggs, often served on sushi, that you can buy at Asian grocery markets. I actually recommend that you eat both fish eggs AND liver, both are exceptionally nutritious foods. This is because fish roe isn't going to be the best source of iron like liver is, so it is best to eat both fish eggs and liver.

Did You Know.....Eating Liver Helps Your Hormones

Liver organ meat is the most nutritious food on the planet. Its exceptionally high vitamin content is relevant to all of your hormones. In the next table, by each nutrient name, you will see how this nutrient helps promote balanced hormones. While you certainly can piece together other foods and supplements to get these nutrients, I suggest that you try incorporating liver into your diet for at least 2 months and see how you feel.

Also, for the following nutrient values in liver, keep in mind that the Daily Value (DV) established by the government are antiquated and these Daily Values don't take into account your period losses or other reasons you might lose nutrients, such as exercise losses, gut issues, and things like prescription-related nutrient losses.

* * *

A 3-4 ounce serving of liver contains:

- **Vitamin B12**: 21 mcg (800% DV). Vitamin B12 is a cofactor in making hormones and hemoglobin. An estimated 40% of older adults are at risk for vitamin B12 deficiency. As vegetarian diets become popular, vitamin B12 deficiency is expected to rise. Stomach medications also

deplete vitamin B12.
- **Vitamin A**: 4300 RAE (400% DV). Liver contains retinol form of vitamin A and reduces symptoms of heavy periods or menorrhagia. It is also important for skin integrity, immunity, and to protect cells.[7-8]
- **Folate** 560 mcg (100% DV): Helps make hemoglobin which supplies oxygen to cells and boosts progesterone levels. You should also know that the folate in animal foods is better absorbed than the folate from green vegetables.[9]
- **Vitamin B6**: 0.8 mg (60% DV): Vitamin B6 is also critical for the metabolism of protein, dampens inflammation, also helps make hormone receptors.[10]
- **Vitamin K2**: 92 mcg (77% DV) liver contains vitamin K2, a nutrient that humans don't get enough of. Vitamin K2 functions to protect bone and heart tissue and even may play a role in **mitochondrial** function. Low levels may impair testosterone production.[11]
- **Selenium**: 36 mcg (47% DV): Selenium is an antioxidant mineral that helps maintain normal thyroid levels which means it helps sex hormones too.
- **Iron:** 13 mg (70% DV for adult women): Liver is the richest source of heme iron of any food out there and incredibly important as reviewed above.
- **Zinc:** 4-5 mg (36%DV): Low zinc levels cause abnormal testosterone levels and also reduce other hormones levels. A zinc-rich diet helps make our body's hormones.
- **Copper**: 14 mg (>700% DV): Copper is needed in small amounts in our diet to form red blood cells and enzymes in the body.
- **CoenzymeQ10**: 5-6 mg: Liver is one of the only natural sources of coenzyme Q10 in foods. Coenzyme Q10 is an antioxidant that is also critical for the production of energy in the **mitochondria**. It helps reduce insulin levels in women with PCOS.[12]

The Broccoli Family-Natural Hormone Detoxifiers

The broccoli family of vegetables, also known as Brassica or cruciferous vegetables, have some amazing properties when it comes to helping balance hormones. They contain two very potent compounds called indoles and sulforaphane precursors which we will discuss in some detail because of their powerful effects.

Indoles From Broccoli Neutralize Hormones

Indoles are a type of antioxidant found in all cruciferous veggies and they do something amazing: they have the ability to keep estrogen balance in the body, and more importantly, detoxify the hormone pathways, making estrogens less carcinogenic.[13] These powerful antioxidants from cruciferous vegetables keep insulin and growth factors in check. Both of these factors are part of the complex environment that affects the growth of cancers in general, as well as other diseases of aging like heart disease. The estrogen balance created by broccoli is key because if you recall, estrogen is the driver of many hormonal issues, even certain types of cancer. Let's dive in a little deeper about how all of this works.

Broccoli's indoles also help keep testosterone balance healthy by keeping testosterone from converting into estrogen. The hormonal balancing act of Brassica is thought to be the reason that they reduce the risk of some of the most common kinds of cancer, including colon, prostate, and breast cancer. Indoles in Brassica also reduce the chances of **cervical dysplasia**, and may be helpful in chronic pain situations such as **fibromyalgia**.

Research also shows that indoles support the liver detoxification process by removing excess hormones in the body. Indole also binds to estrogen receptors and helps shift active estrogen (E1) into a more beneficial form (E3).

As reviewed in Chapter 2, high levels of estrone (E1), the driver, are linked to cancers, specifically breast cancer. In contrast, the healthier form of estrogen (E3) is considered "good" and associated with reduced cancer growth. In other words, estrogen as E1 promotes cancer growth whereas indole from broccoli suppresses cancer growth in tissue studies.[14] Simply put, our bodies make more of a healthier form of estrogen known as E3 when we eat broccoli or any Brassica vegetable.[15]

According to the National Cancer Institute, the estimated number of breast cancer cases in the United States for 2021 is 281,550 in women and 2,650 cases in men.[16] Eating broccoli family vegetables may help battle the estrogen imbalance and decrease cancer risk in both women and men. A study with more than 800 women found that eating cruciferous vegetables, particularly broccoli, reduced breast cancer risk in premenopausal women.[17]

The potent indole from broccoli does another powerful thing: it decreases an enzyme in the body called **aromatase** which converts testosterone to estrogen.[18] This is good because excess aromatase leads to excess estrogen, also known as estrogen dominance. And estrogen dominance can lead to a cascade of unwanted hormonal symptoms.[19] In this case, broccoli is definitely medicine when it comes to PCOS and other hormonal conditions, such as the issue I struggled with, my own issue I used to have called **Mittelsmerz**.

* * *

Did You Know...Broccoli Harnesses Estrogen Health

If you think broccoli is great, a very small serving of broccoli sprouts is even more potent. Broccoli sprouts contain between 10-100 times as much of a powerful compound called sulforaphane than regular broccoli does.[20] This compound is brain-protective, helps clear toxins like heavy metals from the body, and helps protect from neurological conditions. But, I think it's a smart idea to eat a variety of broccoli family foods as listed above to help optimize your health.

Sulforaphane in cruciferous foods, especially broccoli sprouts, reduces excess estrogen levels in the body. For me, raw broccoli essentially cured my mid-cycle ovarian pain as I reviewed on page 142! Broccoli foods also enhance antioxidants in the body. If that wasn't enough, sulforaphane from broccoli fights free radicals produced by UV rays, food additives, and preservatives.[21] You should know that when it comes to sulforaphane, a little goes a long way. A couple tablespoons of broccoli sprouts is a powerful dose of sulforaphane!

You can add radish to any broccoli family of foods to increase its sulforaphane content. Eat your broccoli raw or lightly steam or stir fry your vegetables for no more than 2 minutes because boiled broccoli has no sulforaphane or indoles due to the high temperature of the water. You can also add mustard seed to any broccoli family of foods to enhance its sulforaphane content. For about a half pound (200 g) of broccoli, 1 gram of mustard powder increases the body's levels of sulforaphane by 4 times. Also, eat meat with broccoli foods to increase the absorption of sulforaphane.

Chapter 3

Broccoli Family of Foods That Help Balance Estrogen

The following foods are great to include in your diet to help your body neutralize and balance estrogen when needed:

- Broccoli sprouts (richest in sulforaphane)
- Brussel Sprouts (richest in indoles)
- Garden Cress
- Mustard Greens
- Turnip
- Kale
- Kohlrabi
- Red Cabbage
- Broccoli
- Horseradish
- Cauliflower
- Bok Choy

While Brussels sprouts lead the pack for indoles, almost all cruciferous vegetables will give your body an indole and sulforaphane boost. A common complaint is gas and bloating from broccoli foods, but I contend that this is often related to a leaky gut. By following gut healing principles first, most people can incorporate broccoli foods into their diet with ease. Still, some people may never tolerate broccoli. If this is you, you could consider supplementing broccoli extracts which are readily available on the market today. Or you can try adding a broad-spectrum digestive enzyme supplement such as Seeking Health Digestive Enzymes.

※ ※ ※

Did You Know....Fermented Foods are Friendly Hormone Detoxifiers

Having a healthy gut is an unsung hero of healthy hormones for many reasons: you absorb your food better for one, but did you know that gut bacteria help to neutralize and activate hormones like estrogen when your body is in need? This is in part because a healthy **microbiome** *in the gut helps to produce the enzyme called* **beta-glucuronidase.** *This enzyme helps estrogen in our body to become active, which is a good thing for hormone balance. But you may be confused like you should be because isn't' too much active estrogen bad? Yes. But a healthy gut helps balance the beta-glucuronidase too.*

When there is a gut imbalance there's too little or too much beta-glucuronidase. These imbalances can lead to an excess or deficiency of estrogen in the body.[22] To assure that your body gets a balance of estrogen from the microbiome, make sure to eat fermented foods like raw sauerkraut, fermented vegetables, plain whole milk yogurt, plain kefir, kimchi, and other fermented foods. If these foods are out of the question for your taste palate, you should definitely consider taking a probiotic supplement.

* * *

Gut Balance from Probiotics is Central to Hormonal Balance

In addition to all of the nutrient-rich foods we discussed above, it is important to help improve the health of your gut for hormone balance. Here are some simple tips that will get you started:

Choose whole foods grown in healthy regenerative soil because healthy bacteria feed on certain foods we eat and grow, in turn, make our hormones healthier. Our gut epithelial cells regenerate every 5 days! So it is never too late to turn your eating habits around. I encourage you to become familiar with what it means to have healthy soil and why it is so important for you and for the planet.

Try a broad-spectrum probiotic that contains at least 5 strains of Lactobacillus, Bifidobacterium, and/or Bacillus.

Ditch alcohol and decrease caffeine: we live in a society where a cup of coffee seems to be a must, but our hormones can pay the price. Try a cup of herbal tea or green tea in the morning instead of coffee. Green tea and herbal teas are full of antioxidants, small amounts of caffeine, and estrogen-balancing effects. Alcohol is very toxic to the gut and thus toxic to hormone balance.

Avoid antibiotics when possible: antibiotics alter the gut microbiome and destroy bad and good bacteria. Did you know they also cause you to absorb more heavy metals? Heavy metals are terrible for hormones and your whole body[23].

Eat foods high in fiber: but only choose ones that are tolerable for you. Some people find high-fiber foods cause more pain and disruption for them, especially legumes and grains. Good choices of fiber should be individualized to you as I review in my book Gut Fix. I suggest starting with easy-to-digest fibers like green bananas, oranges, veggie sprouts, berries, and root vegetables.

Kick processed foods to the curb: highly processed foods, including sugar, fast foods, crackers, cookies, cakes, sodas, and the like all cause gut imbalances and thus hormone imbalances. Processed foods also create an imbalance in bacteria which signals our bodies to eat more food, causing cravings, hormonal imbalance, and potential bacterial overgrowth.

Eat plenty of protein foods: as we will soon review, protein is required to support and maintain a healthy microbiome.

Healthy Fats Build Hormones

Wouldn't it be nice if we could think of fats in a simplistic way, as in "all good" or "all bad" as experts thought of them back in the 80s or 90s? It turns out that fats are extremely complex in our foods and so are their effects in our bodies when it comes to hormonal balance and periods.

And what we still are taught as good and bad fats isn't necessarily true when it comes to mainstream media and teaching in higher level education. For example, our bodies need cholesterol to make all of our sex hormones and thyroid hormones. Without adequate cholesterol and saturated fat, some hormones can suffer.

Many women who switch to a higher-fat diet that is high in quality fats while reducing carbohydrate intake enjoy a wonderful improvement in mood and hormonal shifts. This is because healthy fats are the building blocks of cells and hormones.

In fact, natural fats with cholesterol help increase estrogen production naturally and improve good cholesterol [60]. Here is another interesting fact: women who eat more dairy products, rich in saturated fat and cholesterol, enjoy less period pain than those who do not. These women with less period pain eat around 4 servings of full-fat dairy per day.[24]

* * *

Did You Know....Omega 3 Fats Reduce Menstrual Pain

Some kinds of fats, like the ones found in fish and cod liver oil, help reduce menstrual pain too. In fact, fish oil supplements work better than ibuprofen if taken consistently over several months. Now that's some powerful natural medicine! Not to mention, ibuprofen can harm the kidneys if taken frequently over the years. All the while fish oil intake is related to a lower risk of getting kidney disease.[25] Pretty neat, wouldn't you say?

It can't be said enough, eating plenty of fish should be a cornerstone to every diet. However, I have yet to meet anyone in my 25 years of practice who actually eats enough fish for getting adequate omega 3s. The only way to truly guarantee that you are getting enough healthy fats in your body is by supplementing fish oil. Because cod liver oil is a type of fish oil that naturally contains the hormone-happy vitamin A, I suggest going the cod liver oil route instead of just plain fish oil. Cod liver oil absorbs much better than most fish oil supplements too, so you get more for your money. The best cod liver oil on the market today are the fermented cod liver oils made in the traditional way. Taking a combination of vitamin E along with your fish oil dramatically reduces menstrual pain and works as well or better than ibuprofen according to research. In fact, many studies show this.[26-31]

For vegetarians, flaxseed oil provides some omega-3s but I find it can be very gut-disrupting as I reviewed in detail in my book Gut Fix. If you choose to add flaxseed, I suggest soaking it and fermenting it with a little apple cider vinegar with the mother overnight before eating it to make it easier on the gut. Hemp seed as an omega-3 source is often much easier to tolerate than flax if it is hulled. But it's nearly impossible to get enough omega-3 fats from plants because most people don't efficiently convert plant sources into active omega-3 fats. Still, having some plant omega 3s has some additive benefits for reducing toxic estrogen types in the body. I like walnuts and hemp as plant omega-3 sources personally and because they are easier on the gut than other plant omega-3s for many people. Pasture-raised eggs are another good option.

Besides all this, the American diet is much higher in unhealthy omega-6 fats than ever, so it takes much more omega-3 fats than it used to for us to balance this out[32]. Without even trying, people get these inflammatory omega-6 fats by eating chips, crackers, cakes, cookies, pies, fried foods, and the like.[33] If you truly analyze your diet, I'm sure you will find sunflower oil, soybean oil, and other unhealthy fats that disrupt healthy fats. But, you should always try to cut back on these packaged and processed fats as a primary goal.

Women with higher total fat intake tend to have higher levels of estrogen and the hormone precursor called DHEA as well, so eating more healthy fats may ease menopause symptoms too.[34]

To help simplify the confusion, here are some healthy fats to include in your diet:

- Walnuts
- Macadamia nuts
- Almonds
- Fatty, cold water fish like salmon, mackerel, sardines
- 100% grass fed beef
- Olives
- Extra-virgin olive oil
- Hemp seeds
- Pasture-raised eggs
- Avocados
- Grass Fed butter or ghee
- Coconut oil, preferably virgin coconut oil

- Lard (yes lard, it's got a healthier fat profile than most fats!)
- Tallow
- Organic grass-fed whole milk yogurt or cheese

Protein: You Need More If You Love Healthy Hormones

Okay, okay, I know these days there is a lot of controversy about protein and types of protein. But, from my clinical experience, I see most people don't eat enough protein in their diets. This is because mainstream media and professional organizations like the American Heart Association have led us all to shirk some of the healthiest protein sources out there for women, such as eggs and meats. The standing that they take is based on exceptionally weak evidence that has since been disputed by many other research trials. The preponderance of messages still get misconstrued, so women end up being hungry because they don't eat enough protein and compensate by eating too many carbs. Women tend to eat more animal protein as they get closer to their periods which indicates that hormonal changes naturally increase our desire for protein-and probably for a good reason.[35]

Too little protein in the diet may lead to low hormones-especially progesterone which is needed for a healthy uterine lining.[36] Too little progesterone can lead to heavy bleeding as reviewed in Chapter 2. Protein also helps make adequate amounts of estrogen[37]. Long term, too little protein can cause your periods to stop altogether, which is dangerous for your overall health.

Protein is very filling-the most filling of all nutrients. Hard stop. If you don't eat enough, you will overeat everything else. This means that your body will surge too much insulin, which drives all of your other hormones out of balance as we reviewed earlier. The classic example of this is PCOS.

Even a burger isn't much protein in most restaurants and fast foods. Visually you will notice that it is mostly bun, which isn't going to fill you up and will just put empty calories in your belly. The best solution in this case is to just eat the burger without a bun. I find that I can make a nice grass fed burger with healthy fats at home with double the size, less calories, and more nutrients for MUCH less cost and the same amount of time as I can hit the drive-through. MUCH healthier too. And your gut will thank you for it. As a bonus, you can make it a burger bowl filled with veggies topped with a tasty burger and extra virgin olive oil on top. Voila! Dinner is done and you have a tasty, healthy meal. See the recipe section in Chapter 10 for an easy burger bowl recipe.

What about meat and cancer risk? Eating fresh meat isn't even clearly a risk for cancer- far from it-according to research. It all goes back to insulin-like growth factor (IGF-1), which can increase cancer risk and protein can drive up IGF-1. But, you know what also drive up IGF-1? Exercise, especially strength training and no one is claiming that exercise is bad for you. One thing you can easily do to help reduce IGF-1 and cancer risk is gentle **intermittent fasting**, which in and of itself dramatically reduces the risk of cancer. You can review how to intermittently fast on page 165. In other words, animal protein gets a bad rap for no good reason in most cases.

A note about soy and plant-based proteins: sadly, 98% of soy foods today have been heavily sprayed with a chemical called glyphosate (Roundup). Many other plant-based crops have this issue, including wheat and many grains. This chemical, at least in animal studies, causes a reduction of the mature ovarian egg follicles, closed or empty egg follicles, and fibrosis which is a thickening or scarring in the uterus. While we wait for human studies, I personally recommend avoiding soy unless organic if you want healthy hormones and organs.

I found research that showed that soy foods like tofu contain 4 mg of hormone-disrupting chemical called glyphosate per pound of soy.[38] This isn't a small amount; it is a higher amount than you might take for some medications! Much of the beans are also heavily sprayed with chemicals. The take-home message here is that if you are going to get plant-based proteins, make absolutely sure that you are choosing organically grown ones. While soy may be beneficial for reducing breast cancer risk in postmenopausal years, please do choose carefully and make sure it all is organic. Countries where soy intake remains popular have seen a dramatic increase in breast cancer risk, such as China.

So, soy isn't the absolute preventative option for breast cancer that people once thought. Some experts state that the intake of soy is actually higher in the United States than it is in places like China, which is likely due to farm subsidies of soy crops in the US.[39] In China, a larger intake of soy is related to a higher prevalence of obesity too.[40] Last but not least, hormone precursors (DHEA) are lower in women when they eat soy. Interestingly, the opposite happens in men: more hormone precursors with soy than not.[41]

To get enough protein, it is smart to aim for at least 1 gram per kg of body weight or at least 0.43 grams of protein per pound of body weight. So for example, if you weigh 170 lbs, this translates to 73 grams of protein per day or around 7-8 ounces of high-quality protein foods per day.[42]

Carbohydrates-Hormone Friend or Foe?

Insulin is the hormone largely responsible for handling carbohydrates in the body. Sadly, excess insulin, caused by too many carbohydrates in the diet, is rampant among women and can create some other hormonal issues for us. Too much insulin increases testosterone in the body, which gives many women PCOS symptoms, such as irregular periods, facial hair, and other metabolic problems.[43]

Hormonal acne and other conditions are likely also driven by excess carbs in the diet, especially refined sugars. By reducing overall junky carbohydrate intake, many women can help fix a lot of their hormonal issues according to the latest research.[44]

However, healthy carbohydrates are still important in the diet, such as nuts, vegetables, and fruits. For women, the important thing to remember about carbs is to limit or avoid added sugars, sweetened beverages, candies, energy drinks, and desserts. This means you, too, Pumpkin Spice Latte! Processed grains, which means most bread, pasta, and cereals should usually be skipped too. The verdict is still out on whole grains and hormones, but recent research sadly indicates that whole grains may actually increase the risk of breast cancer, often a hormonal-driven disease.[45] While not all research agrees with this, whole grains likely don't help hormonal-driven cancers, especially in this world of carbohydrate excess.[46]

Additionally, 95% of celiac disease, which is an autoimmune disease that is rooted in grain-related gluten, remains undiagnosed. Many people with gluten sensitivity also eat gluten and don't know the damages that they are causing their bodies. Gluten is a hormone disruptor for the thyroid and likely for other hormones too. In fact, women who have thyroid antibodies as is the case with **Hashimoto's thyroiditis**, can enjoy less antibodies if they follow a gluten free diet.[47] As you recall from Chapter 2, having healthy thyroid levels is central to healthy periods too. This is because thyroid diseases are related to gluten intolerance.[48]

So, back to the original question of whole grains. Sure, they can have some healthy components, but you should choose wisely. The threshold to eliminate gluten-containing grains should be low. These grains include wheat, barley, rye, and some oats. And wheat is in almost absolutely everything so you will naturally eliminate most junk by eliminating wheat too, which is a nice side benefit of going gluten-free. Just make sure not to substitute gluten-free junk food for gluten and eat whole foods instead.

Sounds complicated, I know. Don't worry, in the meal planning and recipe section, I will give you plenty of easy ways to lower your carb intake and eliminate gluten without feeling deprived or hungry.

Calcium Should Come From Your Diet

Calcium is worth mentioning when it comes to hormones because it can promote restful sleep. In turn, a good night's rest helps to promote balanced hormones. Not only is calcium good for sleep, it also helps reduce the pain related to periods.

This healthy nutrient is one that can and should come almost exclusively from your diet. By choosing organic, grass-fed dairy sources, sardines, bone broth, and calcium-rich vegetables like broccoli and kale, you should be able to easily meet your calcium requirements. Bear in mind that the calcium from non-dairy milk sources, such as almond milk and soy milk, doesn't absorb well-at all- according to recent research.[49] Plus, the non-dairy milks don't have much protein to speak of either.

Taking calcium supplements can throw off the balance of other minerals like zinc and magnesium, so if you do supplement calcium, do so in a way that is balanced with these other minerals. This gets complicated because most calcium-magnesium-zinc supplements are fraught with problems-they contain poorly-absorbed magnesium in the form of magnesium oxide. So, supplementing calcium can take some careful planning and lots of pills. Here's what it would take: calcium citrate, plus magnesium glycinate, plus zinc gluconate. Don't buy the mineral combinations-they just aren't great for absorption.

By eating calcium-rich foods, you get a natural balance of optimally absorbed zinc and magnesium too.[50] Last but not least, too much calcium from calcium supplements interferes with magnesium and may increase the risk of blood clots.[51-52]

Chapter 3 References

1. Najafi N, Khalkhali H, Moghaddam Tabrizi F, Zarrin R. Major dietary patterns in relation to menstrual pain: a nested case control study. BMC Womens Health. 2018 May 21;18(1):69. https://www.ncbi.nlm.nih.gov/pmc/articles/PMC5963185/
2. Najafi N, Khalkhali H, Moghaddam Tabrizi F, Zarrin R. Major dietary patterns in relation to menstrual pain: a nested case control study. BMC Womens Health. 2018 May 21;18(1):69. https://pubmed.ncbi.nlm.nih.gov/32040961/
3. Krysiak R, Kowalska B, Żmuda W, Okopień B. The effect of ezetimibe-statin combination on steroid hormone production in men with coronary artery disease and low cholesterol levels. Pharmacol Rep. 2015 Apr;67(2):305-9. https://pubmed.ncbi.nlm.nih.gov/25712655/
4. Oluleye OW, Kronmal RA, Folsom AR, Vaidya DM, Ouyang P, Duprez DA, Dobs AS, Yarmohammadi H, Konety SH. Association Between Statin Use and Sex Hormone in the Multi-Ethnic Study of Atherosclerosis Cohort. J Clin Endocrinol Metab. 2019 Oct 1;104(10):4600-4606. https://www.ncbi.nlm.nih.gov/pmc/articles/PMC6736052/
5. Soliman GA. Dietary Cholesterol and the Lack of Evidence in Cardiovascular Disease. Nutrients. 2018 Jun 16;10(6):780 https://www.ncbi.nlm.nih.gov/pmc/articles/PMC6024687/
6. Razaitis, L. The Liver Files. Weston Price. July 2005. https://www.westonaprice.org/health-topics/food-features/the-liver-files/
7. Livdans-Forret AB, Harvey PJ, Larkin-Thier SM. Menorrhagia: a synopsis of management focusing on herbal and nutritional supplements, and chiropractic. J Can Chiropr Assoc. 2007 Dec;51(4):235-46. https://www.ncbi.nlm.nih.gov/pmc/articles/PMC2077876/
8. Borel P, Desmarchelier C. Genetic Variations Associated with Vitamin

A Status and Vitamin A Bioavailability. Nutrients. 2017 Mar 8;9(3):246 https://www.ncbi.nlm.nih.gov/pmc/articles/PMC5372909/

9. Gaskins AJ, Mumford SL, Chavarro JE, Zhang C, Pollack AZ, Wactawski-Wende J, Perkins NJ, Schisterman EF. The impact of dietary folate intake on reproductive function in premenopausal women: a prospective cohort study. PLoS One. 2012;7(9):e46276 https://pubmed.ncbi.nlm.nih.gov/23050004/

10. Oka T. Modulation of gene expression by vitamin B6. Nutr Res Rev. 2001 Dec;14(2):257-66. https://pubmed.ncbi.nlm.nih.gov/19087426/

11. Au NT, Ryman T, Rettie AE, Hopkins SE, Boyer BB, Black J, Philip J, Yracheta J, Fohner AE, Reyes M, Thornton TA, Austin MA, Thummel KE. Dietary Vitamin K and Association with Hepatic Vitamin K Status in a Yup'ik Study Population from Southwestern Alaska. Mol Nutr Food Res. 2018 Feb;62(3):10.1002/mnfr.201700746. https://www.ncbi.nlm.nih.gov/pmc/articles/PMC5803412/

12. Izadi A, Ebrahimi S, Shirazi S, Taghizadeh S, Parizad M, Farzadi L, Gargari BP. Hormonal and Metabolic Effects of Coenzyme Q10 and/or Vitamin E in Patients With Polycystic Ovary Syndrome. J Clin Endocrinol Metab. 2019 Feb 1;104(2):319-327 https://pubmed.ncbi.nlm.nih.gov/30202998/

13. Auborn KJ, Fan S, Rosen EM, Goodwin L, Chandraskaren A, Williams DE, Chen D, Carter TH. Indole-3-carbinol is a negative regulator of estrogen. J Nutr. 2003 Jul;133(7 Suppl):2470S-2475S. https://pubmed.ncbi.nlm.nih.gov/12840226/

14.] Nandini DB, Rao RS, Deepak BS, Reddy PB. Sulforaphane in broccoli: The green chemoprevention!! Role in cancer prevention and therapy. J Oral Maxillofac Pathol. 2020 May-Aug;24(2):405. https://www.ncbi.nlm.nih.gov/pmc/articles/PMC7802872/

15. Thomson CA, Ho E, Strom MB. Chemopreventive properties of 3,3'-diindolylmethane in breast cancer: evidence from experimental and human studies. Nutr Rev. 2016 Jul;74(7):432-43 https://www.ncbi.nlm.nih.gov/pmc/articles/PMC5059820/

16. Breast Cancer Facts and Statistics. Breast Cancer Organization. https://www.breastcancer.org/symptoms/understand_bc/statistics
17. Lin T, Zirpoli GR, McCann SE, Moysich KB, Ambrosone CB, Tang L. Trends in Cruciferous Vegetable Consumption and Associations with Breast Cancer Risk: A Case-Control Study. Curr Dev Nutr. 2017 Jul 18;1(8):e000448. https://www.ncbi.nlm.nih.gov/pmc/articles/PMC5998357/
18. Rajoria S, Suriano R, Parmar PS, Wilson YL, Megwalu U, Moscatello A, Bradlow HL, Sepkovic DW, Geliebter J, Schantz SP, Tiwari RK. 3,3'-diindolylmethane modulates estrogen metabolism in patients with thyroid proliferative disease: a pilot study. Thyroid. 2011 Mar;21(3):299-304.]https://www.ncbi.nlm.nih.gov/pmc/articles/PMC3048776/
19. Rajoria S, Suriano R, Parmar PS, Wilson YL, Megwalu U, Moscatello A, Bradlow HL, Sepkovic DW, Geliebter J, Schantz SP, Tiwari RK. 3,3'-diindolylmethane modulates estrogen metabolism in patients with thyroid proliferative disease: a pilot study. Thyroid. 2011 Mar;21(3):299-304. https://www.ncbi.nlm.nih.gov/pmc/articles/PMC3048776/
20. Yagishita Y, Fahey JW, Dinkova-Kostova AT, Kensler TW. Broccoli or Sulforaphane: Is It the Source or Dose That Matters? Molecules. 2019 Oct 6;24(19):3593. https://www.ncbi.nlm.nih.gov/pmc/articles/PMC6804255/
21. Cao S, Wang L, Zhang Z, Chen F, Wu Q, Li L. Sulforaphane-induced metabolomic responses with epigenetic changes in estrogen receptor positive breast cancer cells. FEBS Open Bio. 2018 Nov 14;8(12):2022-2034. https://www.ncbi.nlm.nih.gov/pmc/articles/PMC6275259/
22. Kwa M, Plottel CS, Blaser MJ, Adams S. The Intestinal Microbiome and Estrogen Receptor-Positive women's Breast Cancer. J Natl Cancer Inst. 2016 Apr 22;108(8):djw029 https://www.ncbi.nlm.nih.gov/pmc/articles/PMC5017946/
23. Ajayi OO, Charles-Davies MA, Arinola OG. Progesterone, selected heavy metals and micronutrients in pregnant Nigerian women with

a history of recurrent spontaneous abortion. Afr Health Sci. 2012 Jun;12(2):153-9. https://www.ncbi.nlm.nih.gov/pmc/articles/PMC3462535/
24. Kesteloot H, Sasaki S. On the relationship between nutrition, sex hormones and high-density lipoproteins in women. Acta Cardiol. 1993;48(4):355-63. https://pubmed.ncbi.nlm.nih.gov/8212969/
25. Abdul-Razzak KK, Ayoub NM, Abu-Taleb AA, Obeidat BA. Influence of dietary intake of dairy products on dysmenorrhea. J Obstet Gynaecol Res. 2010 Apr;36(2):377-83. https://pubmed.ncbi.nlm.nih.gov/20492391/
26. Liu M, Ye Z, Yang S, Zhang Y, Wu Q, Zhou C, He P, Zhang Y, Hou F, Qin X. Habitual Fish Oil Supplementation and Incident Chronic Kidney Disease in the UK Biobank. Nutrients. 2022 Dec 21;15(1):22. doi: 10.3390/nu15010022. PMID: 36 https://pubmed.ncbi.nlm.nih.gov/36615681/
27. Sayon-Orea C, Martinez-Gonzalez MA, Gea A, Flores-Gomez E, Basterra-Gortari FJ, Bes-Rastrollo M. Consumption of fried foods and risk of metabolic syndrome: the SUN cohort study. Clin Nutr. 2014 Jun;33(3):545-9. https://pubmed.ncbi.nlm.nih.gov/23954218/
28. Lin YS, Lu SY, Wu HP, Chang CF, Chiu YT, Yang HT, Chao PM. Is frying oil a dietary source of an endocrine disruptor? Anti-estrogenic effects of polar compounds from frying oil in rats. Ecotoxicol Environ Saf. 2019 Mar;169:18-27. https://pubmed.ncbi.nlm.nih.gov/30412894/
29. Wang R, Deng X, Ma Q, Ma F. Association between acrylamide exposure and sex hormones among premenopausal and post-menopausal women: NHANES, 2013-2016. J Endocrinol Invest. 2023 Aug;46(8):1533-1547. https://pubmed.ncbi.nlm.nih.gov/36602706/
30. Yokoyama E, Takeda T, Watanabe Z, Iwama N, Satoh M, Murakami T, Sakurai K, Shiga N, Tatsuta N, Saito M, Tachibana M, Arima T, Kuriyama S, Metoki H, Yaegashi N. Association of fish intake with menstrual pain: A cross-sectional study of the Japan Environment and Children's Study. PLoS One. 2022 Jul 21;17(7):e0269042. https://pubmed.ncbi.nlm.nih.gov/35862448/

31. Mehrpooya M, Eshraghi A, Rabiee S, Larki-Harchegani A, Ataei S. Comparison the Effect of Fish-Oil and Calcium Supplementation on Treatment of Primary Dysmenorrhea. Rev Recent Clin Trials. 2017;12(3):148-153. https://pubmed.ncbi.nlm.nih.gov/28356030/
32. Zafari M, Behmanesh F, Agha Mohammadi A. Comparison of the effect of fish oil and ibuprofen on treatment of severe pain in primary dysmenorrhea. Caspian J Intern Med. 2011 Summer;2(3):279-82 https://www.ncbi.nlm.nih.gov/pmc/articles/PMC3770499/
33. Wu CC, Huang MY, Kapoor R, Chen CH, Huang YS. Metabolism of omega-6 polyunsaturated fatty acids in women with dysmenorrhea. Asia Pac J Clin Nutr. 2008;17 Suppl 1:216-9. https://pubmed.ncbi.nlm.nih.gov/18296341/
34. Nagata C, Nagao Y, Shibuya C, Kashiki Y, Shimizu H. Fat intake is associated with serum estrogen and androgen concentrations in postmenopausal Japanese women. J Nutr. 2005 Dec;135(12):2862-5. https://pubmed.ncbi.nlm.nih.gov/16317133/
35. Gorczyca AM, Sjaarda LA, Mitchell EM, Perkins NJ, Schliep KC, Wactawski-Wende J, Mumford SL. Changes in macronutrient, micronutrient, and food group intakes throughout the menstrual cycle in healthy, premenopausal women. Eur J Nutr. 2016 Apr;55(3):1181-8. https://www.ncbi.nlm.nih.gov/pmc/articles/PMC6257992/
36. Gupta SR, Anand BK. Effect of protein deficiency on plasma progesterone levels during the menstrual cycle of adult rhesus monkeys. Endocrinology. 1971 Sep;89(3):652-8. https://pubmed.ncbi.nlm.nih.gov/4998467/
37. Biro FM, Summer SS, Huang B, Chen C, Benoit J, Pinney SM. The Impact of Macronutrient Intake on Sex Steroids During Onset of Puberty. J Adolesc Health. 2022 Mar;70(3):483-487. https://pubmed.ncbi.nlm.nih.gov/34836804/
38. Bøhn T, Cuhra M, Traavik T, Sanden M, Fagan J, Primicerio R. Compositional differences in soybeans on the market: glyphosate accumulates in Roundup Ready GM soybeans. Food Chem. 2014 Jun 15;153:207-15. https://pubmed.ncbi.nlm.nih.gov/24491722/

39. Wu AH, Stanczyk FZ, Seow A, Lee HP, Yu MC. Soy intake and other lifestyle determinants of serum estrogen levels among postmenopausal Chinese women in Singapore. Cancer Epidemiol Biomarkers Prev. 2002 Sep;11(9):844-51. https://pubmed.ncbi.nlm.nih.gov/12223428/
40. Wang, X.; He, T.; Xu, S.; Li, H.; Wu, M.; Lin, Z.; Huang, F.; Zhu, Y. Soy Food Intake Associated with Obesity and Hypertension in Children and Adolescents in Guangzhou, Southern China. *Nutrients* **2022**, *14*, 425. https://www.mdpi.com/2072-6643/14/3/425
41. Goldin BR, Brauner E, Adlercreutz H, Ausman LM, Lichtenstein AH. Hormonal response to diets high in soy or animal protein without and with isoflavones in moderately hypercholesterolemic subjects. Nutr Cancer. 2005;51(1):1-6 https://pubmed.ncbi.nlm.nih.gov/15749623/
42. Coelho-Junior HJ, Marzetti E, Picca A, Cesari M, Uchida MC, Calvani R. Protein Intake and Frailty: A Matter of Quantity, Quality, and Timing. Nutrients. 2020 Sep 23;12(10):2915. https://pubmed.ncbi.nlm.nih.gov/32977714/
43. Haffner SM, Katz MS, Stern MP, Dunn JF. The relationship of sex hormones to hyperinsulinemia and hyperglycemia. Metabolism. 1988 Jul;37(7):683-8. https://pubmed.ncbi.nlm.nih.gov/3290626/
44. Foley PJ. Effect of low carbohydrate diets on insulin resistance and the metabolic syndrome. Curr Opin Endocrinol Diabetes Obes. 2021 Oct 1;28(5):463-468. https://www.ncbi.nlm.nih.gov/pmc/articles/PMC8500369/
45. Wu H, Kyrø C, Tjønneland A, Boll K, Olsen A, Overvad K, Landberg R. Long-Term Whole Grain Wheat and Rye Intake Reflected by Adipose Tissue Alkylresorcinols and Breast Cancer: A Case-Cohort Study. Nutrients. 2019 Feb 22;11(2):465. https://www.ncbi.nlm.nih.gov/pmc/articles/PMC6412439/
46. Egeberg R, Olsen A, Loft S, Christensen J, Johnsen NF, Overvad K, Tjønneland A. Intake of whole grain products and risk of breast cancer by hormone receptor status and histology among postmenopausal women. Int J Cancer. 2009 Feb 1;124(3):745-50. https://pubmed.ncbi.nlm.nih.gov/19004010/

47. Krysiak R, Szkróbka W, Okopień B. The Effect of Gluten-Free Diet on Thyroid Autoimmunity in Drug-Naïve Women with Hashimoto's Thyroiditis: A Pilot Study. Exp Clin Endocrinol Diabetes. 2019 Jul;127(7):417-422. https://pubmed.ncbi.nlm.nih.gov/30060266/
48. Hakanen M, Luotola K, Salmi J, Laippala P, Kaukinen K, Collin P. Clinical and subclinical autoimmune thyroid disease in adult celiac disease. Dig Dis Sci. 2001 Dec;46(12):2631-5. https://pubmed.ncbi.nlm.nih.gov/11768252/
49. Shkembi B, Huppertz T. Calcium Absorption from Food Products: Food Matrix Effects. Nutrients. 2021 Dec 30;14(1):180. https://www.ncbi.nlm.nih.gov/pmc/articles/PMC8746734/
50. Zarei S, Mohammad-Alizadeh-Charandabi S, Mirghafourvand M, Javadzadeh Y, Effati-Daryani F. Effects of Calcium-Vitamin D and Calcium-Alone on Pain Intensity and Menstrual Blood Loss in Women with Primary Dysmenorrhea: A Randomized Controlled Trial. Pain Med. 2017 Jan 1;18(1):3-13. https://pubmed.ncbi.nlm.nih.gov/27296057/
51. Seelig MS. Interrelationship of magnesium and estrogen in cardiovascular and bone disorders, eclampsia, migraine and premenstrual syndrome. J Am Coll Nutr. 1993 Aug;12(4):442-58. https://pubmed.ncbi.nlm.nih.gov/8409107/
52. Bristow SM, Gamble GD, Stewart A, Horne AM, Reid IR. Acute effects of calcium supplements on blood pressure and blood coagulation: secondary analysis of a randomised controlled trial in post-menopausal women. Br J Nutr. 2015 Dec 14;114(11):1868-74. https://pubmed.ncbi.nlm.nih.gov/26420590/

Four

Chapter 4

How to Choose Dietary Supplements to Strengthen Your Vitality

Most popular supplement companies sell less-than-desirable synthetic vitamins and poorly absorbed minerals. In other words, most supplements that you find on retail shelves really aren't that great. If you want to learn more, I reviewed supplements and how to find high quality ones in depth in my book called Gut Fix.

You want your supplements to come from reputable companies with third-party testing known as certified **Good Manufacturing Practices**. I also suggest going with supplements that are naturally derived and for each nutrient, I will describe how to find natural forms in this chapter. Our bodies aren't tricked by fake vitamins! In fact, synthetic vitamins can do more harm than good for many people.

Another measure of a quality supplement is when it comes from a reputable distributor. Some supplement manufacturers on major distribution sites can have fake products. Fullscript is a better distributor for supplements because all supplements sold there are third-party tested and the supplement brands they carry are all pharmaceutical-grade and vetted out by healthcare providers. For this reason, I suggest asking your healthcare provider that has a Fullscript account to recommend brands and doses. Alternatively you can use my Fullscript account which is https://us.fullscript.com/welcome/hmoretti As a full disclosure, I do make a small amount of affiliate income with this link.

Powerful Iron- The Uterus's Best Friend

I'm mystified by the complete lack of proper education about iron and how it works to help support healthy periods. In fact, iron might be the one nutrient you need the most of all to help prevent abnormal periods.

In an old study published in the Journal of the American Medical Association researching women with heavy and painful periods (menorrhagia), there was a strong link between low iron levels and having more blood loss. To strengthen these findings they gave supplemental iron to these women and 75% of these women had a reduction in bleeding amount after simply receiving iron supplements.[1]

Yet, not one healthcare provider over the span of 20+ years ever told me this. I actually just found this study recently for myself. All told, there is a complete lack of agreement for how to manage iron deficiency among women with heavy periods. In my experience, you need to take iron supplements and keep taking them as long as your periods continue to be heavy. This might mean your whole reproductive life. But the odds are, the iron will actually help reduce the burden of your menstrual cycle, which is a huge win.

And you may be fully unaware that your iron levels are low if your doctor only checks a hemoglobin level for you. Please ask your doctor to check your ferritin levels. Ferritin is the storage form of iron and you can have a very low ferritin with "normal" hemoglobin levels. I was over 40 before anyone offered to check my ferritin levels and I've paid dearly for this over the years because my hemoglobin was "normal." Around half of women with a normal hemoglobin have iron deficiency!

Personally, I have to take iron daily or every other day to get my iron stores to low-normal ferritin levels around 35 ng/ml. If I slack off on taking iron, my levels quickly plummet into the 15 ng/ml range and seem to cause my periods to immediately get heavier and more painful.

I have a theory: I believe that women who start their lives out with heavy periods are iron deficient from the get go and they can never catch up because of the constant losses.

A most common myth that continues to be spread is that you can get enough iron in your diet if you have iron deficiency due to heavy blood loss. This is incorrect. Spinach or green veggies get a reputation for having iron, but they just aren't good sources. Let me explain. Veggies do contain a small amount of iron but the iron that is there is poorly absorbed. Plant sources of iron, also known as non-heme iron, absorb at about 11% at most and under ideal conditions. Absorption can be almost zero if plant iron is present with anti-nutrients or other minerals like calcium.[2] While vitamin C supplements used to be considered helpful for increasing iron absorption, the latest research shows that it doesn't work better than taking iron supplements alone.[3]

Since 1/4 lb of cooked spinach has 3.5 grams of iron, you would only absorb about 0.35 grams of iron at most from spinach, but probably less; this is not even 2% of your daily needs for iron. In contrast, a typical iron supplement will have between 18 mg and 65 mg of iron per capsule or tablet. The smallest dose of iron supplement is going to have over 50 times the amount of iron as a big portion of spinach, in other words.

But, spinach is often healthy for many other reasons so don't get me wrong. It may give you energy because it is rich in magnesium and other nutrients. In contrast, the iron in seafood and meats are absorbed much more readily, but it still isn't a sure bet to replete your iron stores. And red meat, like steak, falls way behind organ meats as a rich source of iron.

When you have your period, you can lose a LOT of iron. At a minimum, each cup of period blood lost is between 110-125 mg of iron. So if you are a heavy bleeder, you could lose over 150 mg of iron with each period. Do you know how much spinach that would take? 104 pounds of spinach! You better start digging into your spinach bowls now, you won't have much more time for anything else. But even women with "normal" periods can run low in iron for obvious reasons: iron-poor diets, gluten intolerance or Celiac disease, and ongoing blood loss.[4]

If you are a woman of reproductive age, have had children, and have a "normal to heavy flow" for a period, you are NOT getting enough iron in your diet, even if you eat meat.

The absorption of iron is a tightly regulated system in our body, and genes affect how much you will or won't absorb as well.[5] In the average person, animal-source, or heme iron, is absorbed 2-3 times as much as from vegetables or plants. That is still only 20-30% absorption of iron from meat. In contrast, in people with iron-overload disorders, 80-100% of the animal form of iron is absorbed.

But the take-home message overall is that if you have a heavy period, you should please consider checking a blood ferritin level and taking iron supplements.[6] It will most likely help reduce your bleeding and shore up your iron stores. General recommendations for iron for women are 18 mg per day, but these general recommendations don't take into account heavy bleeding or other iron absorption issues.

Food Sources of Iron:[7]

- Spices per gram 8-10 mg (0.8-1 mg absorbed, max)
- Duck liver 3 ounces 30 mg (5-10 mg absorbed, max)
- Spirulina 10 grams has 3 mg (0.3 mg absorbed, max)
- Unsweetened chocolate ⅛ cup 4 mg approx (0.4 mg absorbed, max)
- Chlorella 10 grams has 0.63 mg (0.06 mg absorbed, max and that's a ton of chlorella)
- Beef liver 5 mg (1-2 mg absorbed, max)
- Spinach 1 cup raw 1.1 mg (0.1 mg absorbed, max)
- Beef steak 3 ounces 1.4 mg (0.4 mg absorbed, max)

In case you are wondering like I do, iron also plays a role in hormonal health. People with low iron levels have an increased risk of also having low thyroid levels. Low thyroid levels can cause low estrogen and can disturb insulin levels too. And abnormal thyroid can wreck your period either with too much or too little bleeding or disturb the frequency of bleeding.[8]

All told, iron deficiency will make your periods worse and your hormones out of balance. Please don't let iron deficiency go untreated and undiagnosed. Be proactive and ask for your provider to check your ferritin levels.

Last but not least, don't rely on your cast iron skillets to give you enough iron either. I've used a cast iron skillet as my only cooking source for decades and it did nothing to improve my iron levels.

Vitamin A, The Unsung Hero of Hormones

Adding to the list of "I wish I would have known when I was 13" vitamin A is a big one. While admittedly less is known about how vitamin A interacts with hormones and periods, we know that it does. The reason that we know this is because vitamin A helps make steroid hormones as far as the research shows. And that's good enough for me. But when it comes to the uterus and vitamin A, we know a lot more.

Specifically, vitamin A reduces heavy periods. For example, one old study from back in the 1970s showed that low vitamin A levels is a cause of heavy and painful periods.[9] Closing the loop, vitamin A supplements reduced heavy bleeding in 92% of these patients. Why doesn't this get talked about? And why might you be low in vitamin A? First, because of your period; you lose a lot of nutrients because of your period, especially if you have heavy ones.

Here's another reason you could be low in vitamin A: about 40% of the population at a minimum has a gene that makes it so that your ability to turn most plant sources of vitamin A into active vitamin A in the body is impaired.[10] Most people also avoid the best sources of vitamin A from animal sources too which is a shame. These foods are organ meats like liver and cod liver oil. Eggs are a fairly good source of vitamin A too but have only a fraction of the vitamin A that the liver has.

Fermented cod liver oil, a great source of natural vitamin A, also helps the body naturally make estrogen and progesterone.[11]

For people who are squeamish about eating liver, I suggest taking grass-fed beef liver capsules from a reputable company like MK Supplements or Ancestral Supplements.

Alternatively, you can supplement vitamin A, but you need to get it in the form of retinol or retinyl palmitate if you have the vitamin A gene that impairs the conversion of vitamin A like I do. If you don't know your genetics it is best to err on the side of getting vitamin A from animal sources or supplementing retinol, not beta-carotene.

The other nice thing about vitamin A from liver is that it helps prevent iron overload in tissues, while helping the body use copper correctly. And copper is necessary to make thyroid and estrogen in the body.[12]

When it comes to vitamin A supplements, it's safe to take moderate to higher doses for most people as long as you are getting enough of all vitamins. Because of this, I suggest taking an adequate amount of vitamin D, K, E, and B-vitamins as well. I discuss this balance in detail in my book Gut Fix, but simply eating beef or chicken liver gives you an optimal balance of these nutrients. The exception is vitamin D, which should be tested, checked, and supplemented on its own according to your blood levels as reviewed in Chapter 3.

Yes, there is a risk of toxicity from vitamin A supplements or eating liver, but vitamin A toxicity remains exceptionally rare. But if you are pregnant, make sure you run it by your healthcare provider before taking any extra supplements.

Nutrients to Prevent PCOS?

> *Not only are vitamin A and other nutrients helpful for heavy periods, they may also be part of a healthy way to prevent and manage PCOS. Higher levels of nutrients including vitamin B12, vitamin E, vitamin K, vitamin A, and vitamin D levels reduced the chances of getting PCOS.*[13]
>
> *This isn't too surprising because nutrients help regulate hormone levels. Nutrient-rich foods like organ meats, nuts and seeds, spices, herbs, other meats, and sunshine or vitamin D supplements may go a long*

way towards preventing this challenging condition. You can learn more about PCOS and natural preventive strategies in Chapter 6.

Vitamin C: The Unsung Antioxidant

Absolutely every nutrient affects your hormone levels and vitamin C is no exception. This antioxidant nutrient is required to help dampen inflammation in the body. Interestingly, it helps to even reduce thyroid antibody levels in people who have autoimmune thyroid conditions according to some research.[14] By dampening antibody levels, one can assume that it helps the thyroid and you would be right to assume this. Thyroid conditions also come with a lot of inflammation generally. Vitamin C can help dampen the inflammation too.

Cortisol is the robber of other hormones as you may recall. Not surprisingly, vitamin C can help reduce excess cortisol levels in the body according to research in people who have chronic stress.[15] Research also indicates that synthetic hormones reduce vitamin C levels.[16] So this means that all-told, hormone replacement therapy and birth control can indirectly cause more stress and in effect, make your hormones more imbalanced through this route too.

In postmenopausal women, vitamin C helps to restore vascular function in women who have estrogen deficiency by improving blood flow.[40] Another interesting fact about vitamin C is that it may reduce the risk of osteoporosis in postmenopausal women.[16] Intriguingly, vitamin C may reduce the cancer-promoting effects of excess estrogen too although more research is needed.[18]

A really important thing to know is that eating high amounts of carbohydrates also increases your vitamin C requirements. Research shows that a lower carbohydrate diet increases blood vitamin C levels. Coming full circle, vitamin C supplements help to improve glucose control and improve insulin sensitivity (while also promoting weight loss naturally). By doing so, it may help with other hormones as well, including estrogen because all hormones are connected to how our bodies handle glucose. Research also shows that vitamin C increases progesterone levels. Pretty nifty, eh? Vitamin C helps to increase insulin sensitivity and even help with weight loss, all good things when it comes to hormone balance.[19-20]

In summary, one little vitamin can do a whole lot when it comes to hormonal balance. Ideally, you should minimize junky carbs like sugar and white processed grains in your diet to improve your vitamin C levels, you should eat vitamin C-rich foods like citrus fruits, bell peppers, and kiwi, and even add in some supplemental vitamin C to help balance out your hormones around your period. This is because vitamin C increases progesterone levels in women who struggle with luteal phase hormones.[21-27] Vitamin C doses in these research trials typically use between 500-1000 mg of supplemental vitamin C per day. While some internet claims suggest that vitamin C helps your period to start, there isn't any proof of this.

Vitamin D for Balanced Hormones

To say that vitamin D affects, well, everything, isn't an exaggeration. But, the degree it helps your hormones and periods is still a matter of debate. It reduces chronic pain symptoms in many situations, improves body composition, and helps immunity and bone health, but there's a whole lot more to the story because vitamin D impacts thousands of genes in the body in a positive way.

Without a doubt, vitamin D, as the game saver, plays a central role in all hormones too, the science just is lagging. Research does show some pretty powerful things so far about reproduction and vitamin D. For example, vitamin D supplementation to achieve adequate levels reduces the chance of preterm labor and infections in women.[28-29]

Vitamin D supplements also reduce the symptoms of period pain according to a fascinating study; here is what they did. Approximately 5 days before each woman got her period, she received 50,000 IU of vitamin D3 every 8 hours until the onset of her period. This treatment reduced the pain of periods pretty dramatically, especially after month 2 of treatment.[30] Impressively, a review of 8 clinical trials showed that vitamin D reduces the chances of painful periods.[31]

Other really interesting data shows that vitamin D reduces the chances of excess testosterone levels such as that occurring in women PCOS.[32] Along these same lines of benefits of vitamin D, low levels of both estrogen and vitamin D greatly contribute to the risk of **metabolic syndrome**, which essentially means you are more likely to be overweight with high blood pressure and have abdominal fat if you are low in both vitamin D and estrogen.[33] To further support that vitamin D helps keep our body's hormones in balance is that vitamin D helps improve insulin sensitivity according to a 6-month study published in the European Journal of Endocrinology.[34]

Vitamin D supplements also may help reduce blood levels of thyroid antibodies which ultimately backs my theory that vitamin D as calcitriol is a master regulator.[35] In fact, using 50,000 IU of vitamin D per week improved TSH levels in people with low thyroid levels.[36] And last but not least, vitamin D may help make breast cancer treatment more effective than conventional treatment alone.[37]

In a nutshell, most people need to test and treat low vitamin D levels to help optimize their hormone levels, and the dose should be individualized to treat your specific needs, not simply dosed on the RDI because these recommendations are very outdated.

Did You Know.....Betaine for the Brain

Originally discovered in beets, betaine is a powerful antioxidant that also helps to do a lot of things in the body because it donates methyl which is essential for survival. For example, betaine as trimethylglycine (TMG) is good for the liver and hormones because it is an antioxidant that may reduce the buildup of fat in the body where you don't want it. It may help your hormones to be balanced because it reduces toxins, improves gut barrier function, reduces inflammation, decreases plasma homocysteine, and promotes a healthy microbiome.[38] Of note, it is most helpful in people who have MTHFR gene variants which is about 50% of the population. If you don't know your gene status, you can deduce whether you do or not by how you react to betaine. If you have symptom relief in any way when supplementing it, you probably have the MTHFR variant in my experience. I also speculate that people who go vegetarian and have the MTHFR gene feel worse on this type of diet because of the relatively low amounts of methyl in plant foods. But I digress. Maybe vegetarians and vegans benefit from taking betaine the most, but time will tell. Betaine (as TMG) is a compound that is similar to the mood-enhancing nutrient called SAM-e. SAM-e has been clinically proven to help improve mood and reduce anxiety. When Same is combined with betaine, it works even better than alone according to research.[39] Doses of betaine in research range anywhere from 500 mg to 6 grams per day. Starting at a low dose makes sense.

Quercetin: A Multipurpose Food Extract for Women

Although quercetin has been around for a long time in health-conscious circles, it became a household name during the pandemic because it has some great **antiviral** effects. It has so many amazing functions in the body otherwise, such as how it functions as a fantastic natural antihistamine and also helps balance out women's organs by decreasing oxidative stress and improving insulin sensitivity, especially in women who have PCOS. By doing so, insulin resistance is alleviated, and also improve egg quality and pregnancy rate and outcomes among women with this condition in a new study this year.[40]

Fascinatingly, quercetin may even reduce **endometriosis** by reducing estrogen and progesterone binding in endometrial tissue and even in the brain in early research. Luckily, quercetin is a very safe supplement derived from plants like apples and onions. Clinical trials have used doses of 500-1000 mg per day for women's issues and it is very safe at these doses.[41] Like many other dietary supplements, quercetin absorbs better with fat in your meal so take it with a good-sized meal.

You certainly can get small amounts of quercetin from your diet, which you should, but it isn't going to have the same therapeutic effect as supplements in the case of quercetin. For example, I love and eat onions just about every day of my life, but it isn't enough to have the beneficial effects on my allergies that the 500-1000 mg supplement dose of quercetin that I take does. One other important detail: take quercetin or eat quercetin-rich foods like onions, berries, and apples with fat to improve its absorption.[42]

A Few Other Hormone-Worthy Nutrients

You may recall that the research into women's hormones and menstrual periods is still in its infancy at best. But the basis for all structure and function in our body are the building blocks of life-called nutrients!

As I was digging through the research with a fine-toothed comb, there are definitely gaps in what is known and what is unknown about nutrients. So there is much more to the story here than I can present to you. But I'll do my best with what we do know about according to the most updated research.

Just keep in mind that everything is connected. If you are low in any nutrient, your hormones are likely to suffer. Your periods are also likely to suffer. While I couldn't find any direct research about some nutrients, it's important to understand that there is going to be an effect of nutrients on each and every hormonal situation based on the logic of the structural and functional components of nutrients. After all, they fuel each and every process in our bodies!

Powerful Nutrients for Hormones and Nutrient-Disruptors

Nutrients are powerful when it comes to hormone balance. The irony is that hormone replacement therapy and birth control hormones can disrupt your own nutrients and hormones in the following ways. Birth control and hormone replacement therapies deplete the body of key nutrients-a long list of nutrients: vitamin B6, folate, vitamin B2, vitamin B12, vitamin C, and E, and the minerals magnesium, selenium, and zinc are also robbed by birth control.[43-5]. In other words, if you are on these hormones, you absolutely need to focus on your nutrients in a very systematic way or your whole body and hormones will suffer.

Folate may help increase progesterone levels, but folate may have a darker side when given as folic acid.[45] Higher folic acid levels in the blood may increase the risk of some types of breast cancer.[46] This vital nutrient is only likely to cause harm when given as synthetic folate called folic acid. The best way to get folate in the diet is to eat high **bioavailable** folate foods like beef liver and pasture-raised eggs. Also, serve up a lot of deep leafy green veggies to get more folate. But you should know that plant sources of folate don't absorb as well as animal sources of folate. If you are supplementing folate, I suggest using natural varieties like methylfolate or folinic acid.

Vitamin B6 often helps with sleep and thus helps dampen stress and anxiety, making hormones more readily available for production in the body. Using natural vitamin B6 is the safest and most effective form of vitamin B6. The natural form of B6 as pyridoxal-5-phosphate may even reduce the risk of breast cancer.[47-48] And unlike synthetic vitamin B6 (pyridoxine) natural B6 doesn't have the same risk of toxicity.

Zinc isn't just for immune health. This multi-tasking mineral helps promote circulation and even acts like an antioxidant by neutralizing free radicals. One of the ways that zinc may help hormones and periods is by reducing inflammatory compounds in a way that is similar to anti-inflammatory medications without the nasty side effects that those bring. Using zinc helps reduce painful periods too as it turns out. Zinc supplements may also reduce the development of endometriosis and ovarian endometrial cysts.[49] However, if you take zinc long-term, you need to keep in mind that it can interfere with copper absorption, so just make sure to get zinc with copper if you plan on taking it on a daily basis. You can use a zinc dose of around less than 50 mg a day safely without worrying about interfering with copper.[50-51]

Vitamin E supplements reduce pelvic pain due to menstruation and even reduces blood loss during periods according to a couple of studies.[52-53] It likely works because it dampens inflammatory fats in the body. Fascinatingly, when vitamin E is combined with fish oil, it has an even stronger effect at reducing menstrual cramps.[54] Just be careful to choose natural vitamin E (d-alpha tocopherol instead of dl-alpha tocopherol). On the label you might also see natural vitamin E listed as mixed tocopherols. If you are on blood-thinning medicine, make sure to check with your doctor first before taking vitamin E. You don't have to use high doses either. Around 200-400 mg of vitamin E per day is plenty.

Vitamin K2 is the nutrient most well-known for helping regulate blood clotting but it does a whole lot more. It helps keep bones strong, helps balance thyroid hormones, and even helps protect the heart.[55] Most people also don't realize that it helps prevent excess clotting while also promoting essential clotting functions.[56] Because of this, it isn't a big surprise that low vitamin K levels can contribute to excess uterine bleeding. It is essential for women to get enough vitamin K as vitamin K2. Vitamin K2 is the most effective form of vitamin K, which is in a food called natto, but it's hard to find. You can also get small amounts in grass fed beef, butter, organ meats, and cheese, but because almost everyone is low in vitamin K2, I suggest taking a supplement. Another possible benefit of vitamin K2 is that it plays a role in estrogen metabolism, which may be why higher intakes of vitamin K2 are linked to lower cancer risk. And the beauty is there is no known toxicity of vitamin K2 supplements. Just make sure to talk to your healthcare provider before starting vitamin K if you are on a blood thinning medication.

Thiamine (vitamin B1) is a B-vitamin that works as well as ibuprofen for period pain according to research.[57-58] It has **analgesic,** pain-relieving, effects because it helps dampen inflammation and blocks pain transmission signals in nerves. Some research shows that you need 100 mg per day for this purpose. However, it can take up to two months for you to feel a difference, so you need to give it some time to work. Luckily there is no toxicity of taking thiamine, so you can feel safe trying this remedy. Thiamine plus fish oil also enhance each other's pain relief.[59]

Magnesium is a critical nutrient for essentially everything and this includes a healthy period. This is because magnesium is known to reduce insulin resistance, decrease stress, and improve the quality of sleep while also helping reduce period pain, premenstrual syndrome, and postmenopausal symptoms.[60-61] Most people need to supplement magnesium because our food supply is lacking in this mineral more and more due to modern farming practices. Generally, start with a low dose of around 150-200 mg to see if it helps. You can always increase it if it doesn't.

Chromium is unlike other nutrients in that in too high of doses is considered a heavy metal so it can be dangerous if you get too much. But, too little chromium in the body is problematic too in that it can contribute to insulin resistance. The addition of natural hormone replacement therapy can increase your body's chromium levels.[62] Further, combining natural estrogen and chromium in postmenopausal women reduced inflammation and the result was synergistic when given together.[63-64] Chromium supplements at 1000 micrograms of chromium picolinate per day helps reduce PCOS symptoms.[65-66] Most whole foods will give you chromium, so it's probably best in the long term to get most chromium from your diet unless you are using it to help treat PCOS. You can get chromium from all forms of meat, eggs, fish, oats (gluten-free), fruits such as grapes, and brewer's yeast.

L-tyrosine and 5-hydroxytryptophan are natural amino acids that can help boost brain-happy chemicals which are really important to dampen stress and balance hormones. [67-68] L-tyrosine helps to boost dopamine for feelings of motivation and joy while 5-hydroxytryptophan helps to make serotonin for a calm mood and uplifted mood. Ideally, you should get a ratio of 10:1 of L-tyrosine to 5-hydroxytryptophan in supplements. While they may not help everyone, they are nothing short of a miracle for many people, including myself. If I had to pick my top 5 supplements, this combination would be in my top 5. One of my most popular blogs is about L-tyrosine and you can read all about it here: https://thehealthyrd.com/l-tyrosine-changed-my-life-and-it-may-change-yours-too/. I highly suggest that you also check out Dr. Amen's research in this area and you can also get a free trial of his supplements from a website called Brain MD. And no, you can't necessarily get enough of these in your diet because chemicals in foods like glyphosate make it so the body can't correctly use these nutrients in the body. Glyphosate is found in the soil, water, and air, so there is no true escaping it altogether.

Lion's mane mushrooms and other types of mushrooms may benefit hormonal balance. One **preclinical** study showed that Lion's mane mushrooms helped reduce depressive symptoms in menopause.[69] As a bonus, eating Lion's mane mushrooms may help improve your memory too.[70]

Alpha lipoic acid is an antioxidant found in foods and every cell in your body also makes it. Foods with the highest amounts of alpha lipoic acid are organ meats and other types of meats, but it's still relatively small amounts of this compound in these foods. Supplemental alpha lipoic acid has great potential to help many areas of health including neurological health and helps reduce diabetes complications as well as reduce blood sugar levels. Research shows that alpha lipoic acid in doses of 600 mg alongside mefenamic acid (a nonsteroidal anti-inflammatory drug) worked better to reduce menstrual pain than mefenamic acid alone.[71] You should always make sure to take alpha lipoic acid with thiamine or a natural B complex because alpha lipoic acid supplements can reduce your blood vitamin B1 levels. Alpha lipoic acid may also help women with PCOS especially if used with inositol as described on page 74. Almost 86% of women taking both 800 mg of alpha lipoic acid and 2000 mg of myoinositol had restored menstrual regularity.[72] Now those are some powerful effects with almost no risks of side effects. However, occasionally people get some minor indigestion or headaches from taking alpha lipoic acid.

Inositol- A Helpful Nutrient for Insulin Resistance and PCOS

Inositol is a natural compound that many experts consider an essential nutrient because it helps with cell signaling in the body and is found in high concentrations in the brain. This nutrient is often referred to as vitamin B8 and is found in foods like citrus fruits, melons, and nuts. While legumes and grains have inositol, these foods sadly are often heavily sprayed with chemicals and have anti-nutrients in them that disrupt the gut, so I suggest people seek out other food sources or choose only USDA organic forms. You should also know that common dietary habits and lifestyle changes cause our bodies to need more inositol. The factors that increase our body's requirements for inositol include caffeine, sugar, refined carbohydrate intake, insulin resistance, diabetes, increasing age, and antibiotic medications.[73] Sounds like just about everyone these days, right?

If you have PCOS, inositol should be a must-have with eating a healthy diet as I will review with you in Chapter 8. This is because women with PCOS using inositol are 1.8 times more likely to have a normal menstrual cycle than women receiving a placebo in a recent compilation of 8 studies.[74] Additionally, the use of inositol is equal in effectiveness to metformin for its effectiveness on blood sugar control in women with PCOS. Not only that, inositol helps reduce body mass index (BMI), testosterone, and insulin levels.[75] Most studies used myo-inositol for women with PCOS. However, two studies used a ratio of 40:1 myo-inositol to chiro-inositol.[76] One study also found that using chiro-inositol was also effective for PCOS symptoms in lean women[77]. Inositol may even improve fertility better than the drug metformin in women with PCOS.[78] Research shows that using 300-600 mg of chiro-inositol is helpful for women with PCOS and doses of 4000 mg of myo inositol are effective. The other bonus of inositol is that it has little to no side effects other than occasional gas and bloating.

Iodine: A Delicate Balance

> Iodine is a necessary nutrient for proper thyroid function, which is key to all hormone balance. Too much and too little iodine can be a problem for your thyroid and hormone health, with low levels of iodine causing low thyroid function, and high levels related to thyroid antibodies.[79]

> While there is still debate about the optimal amount of iodine intake, a good way to assure you are getting enough iodine is to get a high-quality

multivitamin with minerals in it. Some experts in the field suggest that 50-250 micrograms per day of iodine is a good amount of daily iodine intake. The RDI is 150 micrograms per day. Some good food sources of iodine in the diet are shellfish and sea vegetables like kelp and nori. While iodized salt is an option, most people eat processed foods these days and packaged foods don't use iodized salt most of the time. This means that if you have been on a packaged foods or restaurant diet for some time, the odds are that you are low in iodine. Still, if you have thyroid antibodies, you may need to actually avoid extra iodine. But here is where it gets confusing: higher iodine intake strongly reduces cancer risk, particularly breast cancer risk, so you may want to weigh the risks versus benefits of more iodine.[80] I believe that if you eat sea vegetables like nori and kelp weekly or bi-weekly, this should satisfy a healthy iodine intake.

Honestly, how much iodine you need really depends on your lifestyle too, because if you are exposed to chlorinated water, fluorine, or bromine, you need more iodine than if you aren't. And most doctors these days aren't going to be checking your iodine status anyway.

Boron-The Unsung Hero of Minerals

Boron is not a boring mineral! This mineral is one that most women (and men) don't get enough of, but they should. Boron helps with proper estrogen and testosterone production and metabolism. Some women enjoy a natural boost in these hormones with boron supplementation if they have baseline low hormone levels.[81] Additionally, boron helps keep bones strong, helps vitamin D work properly, and is also anti-inflammatory while reducing some kinds of pain. While most fruits and vegetables have boron in them, modern farming practices make it so that the foods grown in them don't retain boron well. This means that the food will suffer from low boron too. As a rule of thumb, supplementing boron is safe in doses up to 20 mg per day[82].

Chapter 4 References

1. Taymor ML, Sturgis SH, Yahia C. The Etiological Role of Chronic Iron Deficiency in Production of Menorrhagia. *JAMA*. 1964;187(5):323–327. https://jamanetwork.com/journals/jama/article-abstract/1161803#
2. Gulec S, Anderson GJ, Collins JF. Mechanistic and regulatory aspects of intestinal iron absorption. Am J Physiol Gastrointest Liver Physiol. 2014 Aug 15;307(4):G397-409. https://www.ncbi.nlm.nih.gov/pmc/articles/PMC4137115/
3. Li N, Zhao G, Wu W, et al. The Efficacy and Safety of Vitamin C for Iron Supplementation in Adult Patients With Iron Deficiency Anemia: A Randomized Clinical Trial. *JAMA Netw Open*. 2020;3(11):e2023644. https://jamanetwork.com/journals/jamanetworkopen/fullarticle/2772395
4. Iron Info for Frequent Donations. Red Cross Blood. https://www.redcrossblood.org/donate-blood/blood-donation-process/before-during-after/iron-blood-donation/iron-informationforfrequentdonors.html#
5. Gulec S, Anderson GJ, Collins JF. Mechanistic and regulatory aspects of intestinal iron absorption. Am J Physiol Gastrointest Liver Physiol. 2014 Aug 15;307(4):G397-409. https://www.ncbi.nlm.nih.gov/pmc/articles/PMC4137115/
6. Mansour D, Hofmann A, Gemzell-Danielsson K. A Review of Clinical Guidelines on the Management of Iron Deficiency and Iron-Deficiency Anemia in Women with Heavy Menstrual Bleeding. Adv Ther. 2021 Jan;38(1):201-225. https://pubmed.ncbi.nlm.nih.gov/33247314/
7. Food Data Central. USDA. https://fdc.nal.usda.gov/
8. Luo J, Hendryx M, Dinh P, He K. Association of Iodine and Iron with Thyroid Function. Biol Trace Elem Res. 2017 Sep;179(1):38-44. https://pubmed.ncbi.nlm.nih.gov/28160243/#
9. Lithgow DM, Politzer WM. Vitamin A in the treatment of menorrhagia.

S Afr Med J. 1977 Feb 12;51(7):191-3. https://pubmed.ncbi.nlm.nih.gov/847567/

10. Suzuki M, Tomita M. Genetic Variations of Vitamin A-Absorption and Storage-Related Genes, and Their Potential Contribution to Vitamin A Deficiency Risks Among Different Ethnic Groups. Front Nutr. 2022 Apr 28;9:861619. https://www.ncbi.nlm.nih.gov/pmc/articles/PMC9096837/

11. Macaluso F, Barone R, Catanese P, Carini F, Rizzuto L, Farina F, Di Felice V. Do fat supplements increase physical performance? Nutrients. 2013 Feb 7;5(2):509-24. https://www.ncbi.nlm.nih.gov/pmc/articles/PMC3635209/

12. Vitamin A and Endocrine Health. Biotics Research. https://blog.bioticsresearch.com/vitamin-a-endocrine-health#

13. Shen JY, Xu L, Ding Y, Wu XY. Effect of vitamin supplementation on polycystic ovary syndrome and key pathways implicated in its development: A Mendelian randomization study. World J Clin Cases. 2023 Aug 16;11(23):5468-5478. https://pubmed.ncbi.nlm.nih.gov/37637683/

14. Farasati Far B, Behnoush AH, Ghondaghsaz E, Habibi MA, Khalaji A. The interplay between vitamin C and thyroid. Endocrinol Diabetes Metab. 2023 Jul;6(4):e432. https://www.ncbi.nlm.nih.gov/pmc/articles/PMC10335618/

15. Beglaryan N, Hakobyan G, Nazaretyan E. Vitamin C supplementation alleviates hypercortisolemia caused by chronic stress. Stress Health. 2023 Nov 27. https://pubmed.ncbi.nlm.nih.gov/38010274/

16. Basu TK. Effects of estrogen and progestogen on the ascorbic acid status of women's guinea pigs. J Nutr. 1986 Apr;116(4):570-7. https://pubmed.ncbi.nlm.nih.gov/3958805/

17. McSorley PT, Young IS, Bell PM, Fee JP, McCance DR. Vitamin C improves endothelial function in healthy estrogen-deficient postmenopausal women. Climacteric. 2003 Sep;6(3):238-47. https://pubmed.ncbi.nlm.nih.gov/14567772/

18. Mangano KM, Noel SE, Dawson-Hughes B, Tucker KL. Sufficient

Plasma Vitamin C Is Related to Greater Bone Mineral Density among Postmenopausal Women from the Boston Puerto Rican Health Study. J Nutr. 2021 Dec 3;151(12):3764-3772. https://pubmed.ncbi.nlm.nih.gov/34510185/

19. Liehr JG. Vitamin C reduces the incidence and severity of renal tumors induced by estradiol or diethylstilbestrol. Am J Clin Nutr. 1991 Dec;54(6 Suppl):1256S-1260S. https://pubmed.ncbi.nlm.nih.gov/1962579/

20. Ashor AW, Werner AD, Lara J, Willis ND, Mathers JC, Siervo M. Effects of vitamin C supplementation on glycaemic control: a systematic review and meta-analysis of randomised controlled trials. Eur J Clin Nutr. 2017 Dec;71(12):1371-1380. https://pubmed.ncbi.nlm.nih.gov/28294172/

21. Johnston CS. Strategies for healthy weight loss: from vitamin C to the glycemic response. J Am Coll Nutr. 2005 Jun;24(3):158-65. https://pubmed.ncbi.nlm.nih.gov/15930480/#

22. *Henmi, H., Endo, T., Kitajima, Y., Manase, K., Hata, H., & Kudo, R. (2003). Effects of ascorbic acid supplementation on serum progesterone levels in patients with a luteal phase defect. Fertility and Sterility, 80(2), 459–461.* https://www.fertstert.org/article/S0015-0282(03)00657-5/fulltext

23. Johnstone AM, Lobley GE, Horgan GW, Bremner DM, Fyfe CL, Morrice PC, Duthie GG. Effects of a high-protein, low-carbohydrate v. high-protein, moderate-carbohydrate weight-loss diet on antioxidant status, endothelial markers and plasma indices of the cardiometabolic profile. Br J Nutr. 2011 Jul;106(2):282-91. https://pubmed.ncbi.nlm.nih.gov/21521539/

24. Ashor AW, Werner AD, Lara J, Willis ND, Mathers JC, Siervo M. Effects of vitamin C supplementation on glycaemic control: a systematic review and meta-analysis of randomised controlled trials. Eur J Clin Nutr. 2017 Dec;71(12):1371-1380. https://pubmed.ncbi.nlm.nih.gov/28294172/

25. Szarka A, Lőrincz T. A C-vitamin celluláris, intracelluláris transzportja. Fiziológiai vonatkozások [Cellular and intracellular transport of vita-

26. min C. The physiologic aspects]. Orv Hetil. 2013 Oct 20;154(42):1651-6. Hungarian. https://pubmed.ncbi.nlm.nih.gov/24121217/
26. Will JC, Ford ES, Bowman BA. Serum vitamin C concentrations and diabetes: findings from the Third National Health and Nutrition Examination Survey, 1988-1994. Am J Clin Nutr. 1999 Jul;70(1):49-52. https://pubmed.ncbi.nlm.nih.gov/10393138/
27. Chen L, Jia RH, Qiu CJ, Ding G. Hyperglycemia inhibits the uptake of dehydroascorbate in tubular epithelial cell. Am J Nephrol. 2005 Sep-Oct;25(5):459-65. https://pubmed.ncbi.nlm.nih.gov/16118484/#
28. Bodnar LM, Platt RW, Simhan HN. Early-pregnancy vitamin D deficiency and risk of preterm birth subtypes. Obstet Gynecol. 2015 Feb;125(2):439-447. https://www.ncbi.nlm.nih.gov/pmc/articles/PMC4304969/
29. Bodnar LM, Krohn MA, Simhan HN. Maternal vitamin D deficiency is associated with bacterial vaginosis in the first trimester of pregnancy. J Nutr. 2009 Jun;139(6):1157-61. https://pubmed.ncbi.nlm.nih.gov/19357214/
30. Amzajerdi A, Keshavarz M, Ghorbali E, Pezaro S, Sarvi F. The effect of vitamin D on the severity of dysmenorrhea and menstrual blood loss: a randomized clinical trial. BMC Womens Health. 2023 Mar 27;23(1):138. https://www.ncbi.nlm.nih.gov/pmc/articles/PMC10045437/
31. Chen YC, Chiang YF, Lin YJ, Huang KC, Chen HY, Hamdy NM, Huang TC, Chang HY, Shieh TM, Huang YJ, Hsia SM. Effect of Vitamin D Supplementation on Primary Dysmenorrhea: A Systematic Review and Meta-Analysis of Randomized Clinical Trials. Nutrients. 2023 Jun 21;15(13):2830. https://pubmed.ncbi.nlm.nih.gov/37447156/
32. Chu C, Tsuprykov O, Chen X, Elitok S, Krämer BK, Hocher B. Relationship Between Vitamin D and Hormones Important for Human Fertility in Reproductive-Aged Women. Front Endocrinol (Lausanne). 2021 Apr 14;12:666687. https://pubmed.ncbi.nlm.nih.gov/33935976/

33. Huang H, Guo J, Chen Q, Chen X, Yang Y, Zhang W, Liu Y, Chen X, Yang D. The synergistic effects of vitamin D and estradiol deficiency on metabolic syndrome in Chinese postmenopausal women. Menopause. 2019 Oct;26(10):1171-1177. https://pubmed.ncbi.nlm.nih.gov/31188285/
34. Rasouli N, Brodsky IG, Chatterjee R, Kim SH, Pratley RE, Staten MA, Pittas AG; D2d Research Group. Effects of Vitamin D Supplementation on Insulin Sensitivity and Secretion in Prediabetes. J Clin Endocrinol Metab. 2022 Jan 1;107(1):230-240. https://pubmed.ncbi.nlm.nih.gov/34473295/
35. Chaudhary, Sandeep; Dutta, Deep1; Kumar, Manoj; Saha, Sudipta2; Mondal, Samim Ali3; Kumar, Ashok; Mukhopadhyay, Satinath. Vitamin D supplementation reduces thyroid peroxidase antibody levels in patients with autoimmune thyroid disease: An open-labeled randomized controlled trial. Indian Journal of Endocrinology and Metabolism 20(3):p 391-398, May–Jun 2016. https://journals.lww.com/indjem/fulltext/2016/20030/vitamin_d_supplementation_reduces_thyroid.20.aspx
36. Villa A, Corsello A, Cintoni M, Papi G, Pontecorvi A, Corsello SM, Paragliola RM. Effect of vitamin D supplementation on TSH levels in euthyroid subjects with autoimmune thyroiditis. Endocrine. 2020 Oct;70(1):85-91. https://pubmed.ncbi.nlm.nih.gov/32239452/
37. Santos-Martínez N, Díaz L, Ortiz-Ortega VM, Ordaz-Rosado D, Prado-Garcia H, Avila E, Larrea F, García-Becerra R. Calcitriol induces estrogen receptor α expression through direct transcriptional regulation and epigenetic modifications in estrogen receptor-negative breast cancer cells. Am J Cancer Res. 2021 Dec 15;11(12):5951-5964. https://pubmed.ncbi.nlm.nih.gov/35018235/
38. Kim R, Nijhout HF, Reed MC. One-carbon metabolism during the menstrual cycle and pregnancy. PLoS Comput Biol. 2021 Dec 16;17(12):e1009708. https://www.ncbi.nlm.nih.gov/pmc/articles/PMC8741061/
39. Di Pierro F, Orsi R, Settembre R. Role of betaine in improving the

antidepressant effect of S-adenosyl-methionine in patients with mild-to-moderate depression. J Multidiscip Healthc. 2015 Jan 16;8:39-45. https://www.ncbi.nlm.nih.gov/pmc/articles/PMC4303396/
40. Vaez S, Parivr K, Amidi F, Rudbari NH, Moini A, Amini N. Quercetin and polycystic ovary syndrome; inflammation, hormonal parameters and pregnancy outcome: A randomized clinical trial. Am J Reprod Immunol. 2023 Mar;89(3):e13644. https://pubmed.ncbi.nlm.nih.gov/36317442/
41. Rezvan N, Moini A, Janani L, Mohammad K, Saedisomeolia A, Nourbakhsh M, Gorgani-Firuzjaee S, Mazaherioun M, Hosseinzadeh-Attar MJ. Effects of Quercetin on Adiponectin-Mediated Insulin Sensitivity in Polycystic Ovary Syndrome: A Randomized Placebo-Controlled Double-Blind Clinical Trial. Horm Metab Res. 2017 Feb;49(2):115-121. https://pubmed.ncbi.nlm.nih.gov/27824398/
42. Guo Y, Mah E, Davis CG, Jalili T, Ferruzzi MG, Chun OK, Bruno RS. Dietary fat increases quercetin bioavailability in overweight adults. Mol Nutr Food Res. 2013 May;57(5):896-905. https://pubmed.ncbi.nlm.nih.gov/23319447/
43. Palmery M, Saraceno A, Vaiarelli A, Carlomagno G. Oral contraceptives and changes in nutritional requirements. Eur Rev Med Pharmacol Sci. 2013 Jul;17(13):1804-13. https://pubmed.ncbi.nlm.nih.gov/23852908/
44. Brown RR, Rose DP, Leklem JE, Linkswiler H, Anand R. Urinary 4-pyridoxic acid, plasma pyridoxal phosphate, and erythrocyte aminotransferase levels in oral contraceptive users receiving controlled intakes of vitamin B6. Am J Clin Nutr. 1975 Jan;28(1):10-9. https://pubmed.ncbi.nlm.nih.gov/1115011/
45. Gaskins AJ, Mumford SL, Chavarro JE, Zhang C, Pollack AZ, Wactawski-Wende J, Perkins NJ, Schisterman EF. The impact of dietary folate intake on reproductive function in premenopausal women: a prospective cohort study. PLoS One. 2012;7(9):e46276. https://www.ncbi.nlm.nih.gov/pmc/articles/PMC3458830/
46. Ericson U, Borgquist S, Ivarsson MI, Sonestedt E, Gullberg B, Carlson

J, Olsson H, Jirström K, Wirfält E. Plasma folate concentrations are positively associated with risk of estrogen receptor beta negative breast cancer in a Swedish nested case control study. J Nutr. 2010 Sep;140(9):1661-8. https://pubmed.ncbi.nlm.nih.gov/20592103/
47. Kennedy DO. B Vitamins and the Brain: Mechanisms, Dose and Efficacy—A Review. Nutrients. 2016 Jan 27;8(2):68. doi: 10.3390/nu8020068. https://www.ncbi.nlm.nih.gov/pmc/articles/PMC4772032/
48. Lin J, Lee IM, Cook NR, Selhub J, Manson JE, Buring JE, Zhang SM. Plasma folate, vitamin B-6, vitamin B-12, and risk of breast cancer in women. Am J Clin Nutr. 2008 Mar;87(3):734-43. https://pubmed.ncbi.nlm.nih.gov/18326613/
49. Onuma T, Mizutani T, Fujita Y, Ohgami N, Ohnuma S, Kato M, Yoshida Y. Zinc deficiency is associated with the development of ovarian endometrial cysts. Am J Cancer Res. 2023 Mar 15;13(3):1049-1066. https://pubmed.ncbi.nlm.nih.gov/37034203/
50. Teimoori B, Ghasemi M, Hoseini ZS, Razavi M. The Efficacy of Zinc Administration in the Treatment of Primary Dysmenorrhea. Oman Med J. 2016 Mar;31(2):107-11. https://www.ncbi.nlm.nih.gov/pmc/articles/PMC4861396/
51. Holt RR, Uriu-Adams JY, Keen CL. Zinc. In: Erdman Jr JW, Macdonald IA, Zeisel SH, eds. Present Knowledge in Nutrition. 10th ed. Washington D.C.: ILSI Press; 2012:521-539.
52. Kashanian M, Lakeh MM, Ghasemi A, Noori S. Evaluation of the effect of vitamin E on pelvic pain reduction in women suffering from primary dysmenorrhea. J Reprod Med. 2013 Jan-Feb;58(1-2):34-8. https://pubmed.ncbi.nlm.nih.gov/23447916/
53. Kashanian M, Lakeh MM, Ghasemi A, Noori S. Evaluation of the effect of vitamin E on pelvic pain reduction in women suffering from primary dysmenorrhea. J Reprod Med. 2013 Jan-Feb;58(1-2):34-8. https://pubmed.ncbi.nlm.nih.gov/23447916/
54. Ziaei S, Zakeri M, Kazemnejad A. A randomised controlled trial of vitamin E in the treatment of primary dysmenorrhoea. BJOG. 2005

Apr;112(4):466-9. https://pubmed.ncbi.nlm.nih.gov/15777446/
55. Negrev NN, Radev RZ, Velikova MS, Anogeianaki A. Effects of the hormones of the thyroid axis on the vitamin K-dependent plasma factors of blood coagulation (II, VII, IX, and X). Int J Immunopathol Pharmacol. 2008 Jan-Mar;21(1):221-6. https://pubmed.ncbi.nlm.nih.gov/18336749/
56. Sadeghi N, Paknezhad F, Rashidi Nooshabadi M, Kavianpour M, Jafari Rad S, Khadem Haghighian H. Vitamin E and fish oil, separately or in combination, on treatment of primary dysmenorrhea: a double-blind, randomized clinical trial. Gynecol Endocrinol. 2018 Sep;34(9):804-808. https://pubmed.ncbi.nlm.nih.gov/29542390/
57. Calderon-Ospina CA, Nava-Mesa MO, Arbeláez Ariza CE. Effect of Combined Diclofenac and B Vitamins (Thiamine, Pyridoxine, and Cyanocobalamin) for Low Back Pain Management: Systematic Review and Meta-analysis. Pain Med. 2020 Apr 1;21(4):766-781. https://www.ncbi.nlm.nih.gov/pmc/articles/PMC7139211/
58. Zafari, Mandana & Aghamohammadi, Azar & Tofighi Niaki, Maryam. (2011). Comparing the effect of vitamin B1 (vit. B1) and ibuberofen on the treatment of primary dysmenorhea. African Journal of Pharmacy and Pharmacology. 5. 874-878. https://academicjournals.org/article/article1380796129_Zafari.pdf
59. Hosseinlou A, Alinejad V, Alinejad M, Aghakhani N. The effects of fish oil capsules and vitamin B1 tablets on duration and severity of dysmenorrhea in students of high school in Urmia-Iran. Glob J Health Sci. 2014 Sep 18;6(7 Spec No):124-9. https://pubmed.ncbi.nlm.nih.gov/25363189/
60. Kolanu BR, Vadakedath S, Boddula V, Kandi V. Activities of Serum Magnesium and Thyroid Hormones in Pre-, Peri-, and Post-menopausal Women. Cureus. 2020 Jan 3;12(1):e6554. doi: 10.7759/cureus.6554. https://www.ncbi.nlm.nih.gov/pmc/articles/PMC6996468/
61. Parazzini F et al. Magnesium in the gynecological practice: a literature review. Magnes Res. 2017 Feb 1;30(1):1-7. https://pubmed.ncbi.nlm.nih.gov/28392498/

62. Roussel AM, Bureau I, Favier M, Polansky MM, Bryden NA, Anderson RA. Beneficial effects of hormonal replacement therapy on chromium status and glucose and lipid metabolism in postmenopausal women. Maturitas. 2002 May 20;42(1):63-9 https://pubmed.ncbi.nlm.nih.gov/12020981/
63. Jain SK, Rogier K, Prouty L, Jain SK. Protective effects of 17beta-estradiol and trivalent chromium on interleukin-6 secretion, oxidative stress, and adhesion of monocytes: relevance to heart disease in postmenopausal women. Free Radic Biol Med. 2004 Dec 1;37(11):1730-5. https://pubmed.ncbi.nlm.nih.gov/15528032/
64. Ajayi OO, Charles-Davies MA, Arinola OG. Progesterone, selected heavy metals and micronutrients in pregnant Nigerian women with a history of recurrent spontaneous abortion. Afr Health Sci. 2012 Jun;12(2):153-9. https://www.ncbi.nlm.nih.gov/pmc/articles/PMC3462535/
65. Fazelian S, Rouhani MH, Bank SS, Amani R. Chromium supplementation and polycystic ovary syndrome: A systematic review and meta-analysis. J Trace Elem Med Biol. 2017 Jul;42:92-96. https://pubmed.ncbi.nlm.nih.gov/28595797/
66. Amr N, Abdel-Rahim HE. The effect of chromium supplementation on polycystic ovary syndrome in adolescents. J Pediatr Adolesc Gynecol. 2015 Apr;28(2):114-8. https://pubmed.ncbi.nlm.nih.gov/25850593/
67. van Kessel SP, Frye AK, El-Gendy AO, Castejon M, Keshavarzian A, van Dijk G, El Aidy S. Gut bacterial tyrosine decarboxylases restrict levels of levodopa in the treatment of Parkinson's disease. Nat Commun. 2019 Jan 18;10(1):310. https://www.ncbi.nlm.nih.gov/pmc/articles/PMC6338741/
68. Mouret J, Lemoine P, Minuit MP, Robelin N. La L-tyrosine guérit, immédiatement et à long terme, les dépressions dopamino-dépendantes (DDD). Etude clinique et polygraphique [L-tyrosine cures, immediate and long term, dopamine-dependent depressions. Clinical and polygraphic studies]. C R Acad Sci III. 1988;306(3):93-8. French https://pubmed.ncbi.nlm.nih.gov/3126995/

69. Anuar AM, Minami A, Matsushita H, Ogino K, Fujita K, Nakao H, Kimura S, Sabaratnam V, Umehara K, Kurebayashi Y, Takahashi T, Kanazawa H, Wakatsuki A, Suzuki T, Takeuchi H. Ameliorating Effect of the Edible Mushroom Hericium erinaceus on Depressive-Like Behavior in Ovariectomized Rats. Biol Pharm Bull. 2022;45(10):1438-1443. https://pubmed.ncbi.nlm.nih.gov/36184501/
70. Cha S, Bell L, Shukitt-Hale B, Williams CM. A review of the effects of mushrooms on mood and neurocognitive health across the lifespan. Neurosci Biobehav Rev. 2024 Mar;158:105548. https://pubmed.ncbi.nlm.nih.gov/38246232/
71. Yousefi M, Kavianpour M, Hesami S, Rashidi Nooshabadi M, Khadem Haghighian H. Effect of alpha-lipoic acid at the combination with mefenamic acid in girls with primary dysmenorrhea: randomized, double-blind, placebo-controlled clinical trial. Gynecol Endocrinol. 2019 Sep;35(9):782-786. https://pubmed.ncbi.nlm.nih.gov/30957578/
72. Fruzzetti, F., Benelli, E., Fidecicchi, T., & Tonacchera, M. (2020). Clinical and metabolic effects of alpha-lipoic acid associated with two different doses of myo-inositol in women with polycystic ovary syndrome. *International Journal of Endocrinology, 2020*, 1–8. https://www.hindawi.com/journals/ije/2020/2901393/
73. DAUGHADAY WH, LARNER J. The renal excretion of inositol in normal and diabetic human beings. J Clin Invest. 1954 Mar;33(3):326-32. https://www.ncbi.nlm.nih.gov/pmc/articles/PMC1072508/
74. Greff D, Juhász AE, Váncsa S, Váradi A, Sipos Z, Szinte J, Park S, Hegyi P, Nyirády P, Ács N, Várbíró S, Horváth EM. Inositol is an effective and safe treatment in polycystic ovary syndrome: a systematic review and meta-analysis of randomized controlled trials. Reprod Biol Endocrinol. 2023 Jan 26;21(1):10. https://pubmed.ncbi.nlm.nih.gov/36703143/
75. Benelli E, Del Ghianda S, Di Cosmo C, Tonacchera M. A Combined Therapy with Myo-Inositol and D-Chiro-Inositol Improves Endocrine Parameters and Insulin Resistance in PCOS Young Overweight Women. Int J Endocrinol. 2016;2016:3204083. https://www.

ncbi.nlm.nih.gov/pmc/articles/PMC4963579/
76. Benelli E, Del Ghianda S, Di Cosmo C, Tonacchera M. A Combined Therapy with Myo-Inositol and D-Chiro-Inositol Improves Endocrine Parameters and Insulin Resistance in PCOS Young Overweight Women. Int J Endocrinol. 2016;2016:3204083. https://www.ncbi.nlm.nih.gov/pmc/articles/PMC4963579/
77. Juorno MJ, Jakubowicz DJ, Baillargeon JP, Dillon P, Gunn RD, Allan G, Nestler JE. Effects of d-chiro-inositol in lean women with the polycystic ovary syndrome. Endocr Pract. 2002 Nov-Dec;8(6):417-23. https://pubmed.ncbi.nlm.nih.gov/15251831/
78. Raffone E, Rizzo P, Benedetto V. Insulin sensitiser agents alone and in co-treatment with r-FSH for ovulation induction in PCOS women. Gynecol Endocrinol. 2010 Apr;26(4):275-80. https://pubmed.ncbi.nlm.nih.gov/20222840/
79. Farebrother J, Zimmermann MB, Assey V, Castro MC, Cherkaoui M, Fingerhut R, Jia Q, Jukic T, Makokha A, San Luis TO, Wegmüller R, Andersson M. Thyroglobulin Is Markedly Elevated in 6- to 24-Month-Old Infants at Both Low and High Iodine Intakes and Suggests a Narrow Optimal Iodine Intake Range. Thyroid. 2019 Feb;29(2):268-277. https://pubmed.ncbi.nlm.nih.gov/30648484/
80. Rappaport J. Changes in Dietary Iodine Explains Increasing Incidence of Breast Cancer with Distant Involvement in Young Women. J Cancer. 2017 Jan 13;8(2):174-177. https://www.ncbi.nlm.nih.gov/pmc/articles/PMC5327366/
81. Pizzorno L. Nothing Boring About Boron. Integr Med (Encinitas). 2015 Aug;14(4):35-48. https://www.ncbi.nlm.nih.gov/pmc/articles/PMC4712861/

Chapter 5

Herbs for A Vital and Happy Uterus

Herbs are some of the best and yet unsung heroes of the hormonal world and of reproductive organs. I can tell you countless ways that herbs have kept me off of prescription medications which makes me so happy because these medications gave me terrible side effects! And if you are like me, you will be happy that many herbal therapies come with **side benefits** instead of major side effects in most cases.[1]

Science is beginning to finally understand what indigenous people have known all along-that plants have their own intelligence and are more complex than we give them credit for. I encourage you to take some time to get to know more healing plants by their smell, taste, where they grow, and what they are traditionally used for. It's great to grow some of your own too. After all, medicine used to be based on complex observation. Now it is based on reductionist science which isolates one aspect of health, such as a lab value, but fails to fully understand the human experience together as a whole. I highly recommend that you read the book called *Braiding Sweetgrass* by Robyn Wall Kimmerer to get a deeper understanding of the plant and natural world. While we will never fully understand the communication that these herbs and plants have, by becoming in tune with the natural world around us, we can become more in tune with our own selves and how we relate to everything. Plants have their own intelligence and they will tell you about it if you just listen, observe, and honor traditional uses that are now being proven out by scientific methods.

Still, you should always check with your healthcare provider before changing up your herbal routine. But be aware that medical schools STILL shirk the teaching of herbs, so your conventional doctor isn't going to be a whole lot of help here in most cases. Try seeking out a functional medicine provider or a reputable naturopath that has a deep understanding of herbal remedies to get the most benefits from herbs.

This chapter will help you understand the options available so that you can begin to observe and have a conversation with your provider and establish a plan suited for you as an individual. After all, we are all different, so why should our herbal routines all be the same?

Harmonious Herbs

> *You should know that herbs and natural remedies are quite different from pharmaceuticals. Herbs have their own built-in checks and balances that help promote stability in the body and this doesn't happen with pharmaceuticals. Herbs often have hundreds upon hundreds of beneficial and unique compounds that balance each other out. Sadly, the pharmaceutical world often tries to imitate nature without success. This is because prescription drugs don't have the balance factors that nature gives them like herbs and plants do. For example, prescriptions may be meant to blast out a particular enzyme in the body or completely mask*

your own hormones as is the case of oral contraceptives and hormone replacement therapy.

A good example of an herb with a perfect harmony of checks and balances in place is saffron. This beautiful and delicate herb has over 150 active compounds and has the ability to decrease cortisol hormone, which in effect prevents the "cortisol steal." By doing so, it promotes a feeling of calm and thereby naturally helps promote a balance of estrogen, testosterone, and progesterone. All the while, this potent herb decreases inflammation in the body and also helps reduce cancer risk.[2] As a culinary herb, it is very well tolerated with no known side effects at moderate doses (except if you are allergic, then definitely avoid it). Saffron is effective in reducing PMS symptoms in clinical studies at doses as low as 30 mg per day. In fact, a compilation of 5 clinical studies shows that saffron is effective in helping treat major depression.[3] See Figure 2 for how herbs can help our body in the most holistic way.

I urge you to compare this stack of interesting effects of saffron to the effects and side effects of other prescription medications used for depression or hormones. Prescriptions have one compound and herbs have hundreds of compounds that enhance each other and balance each other. However, I am in no way discouraging the use of antidepressant or hormonal medications, I'm simply pointing out that nature often gets it right when it comes to checks and balances.

Granted, there are times and places where there are side effects to herbal supplements. But, these cases are fewer and farther between than you might think. Herbs have been used since humans have existed on the planet. If there is a major risk, you will know about it because there are case reports all over the news about it. For this book, I'm not including the dangerous herbs or plants that have any big known risks such as ephedra.

Period Fix

* * *

Chapter 5

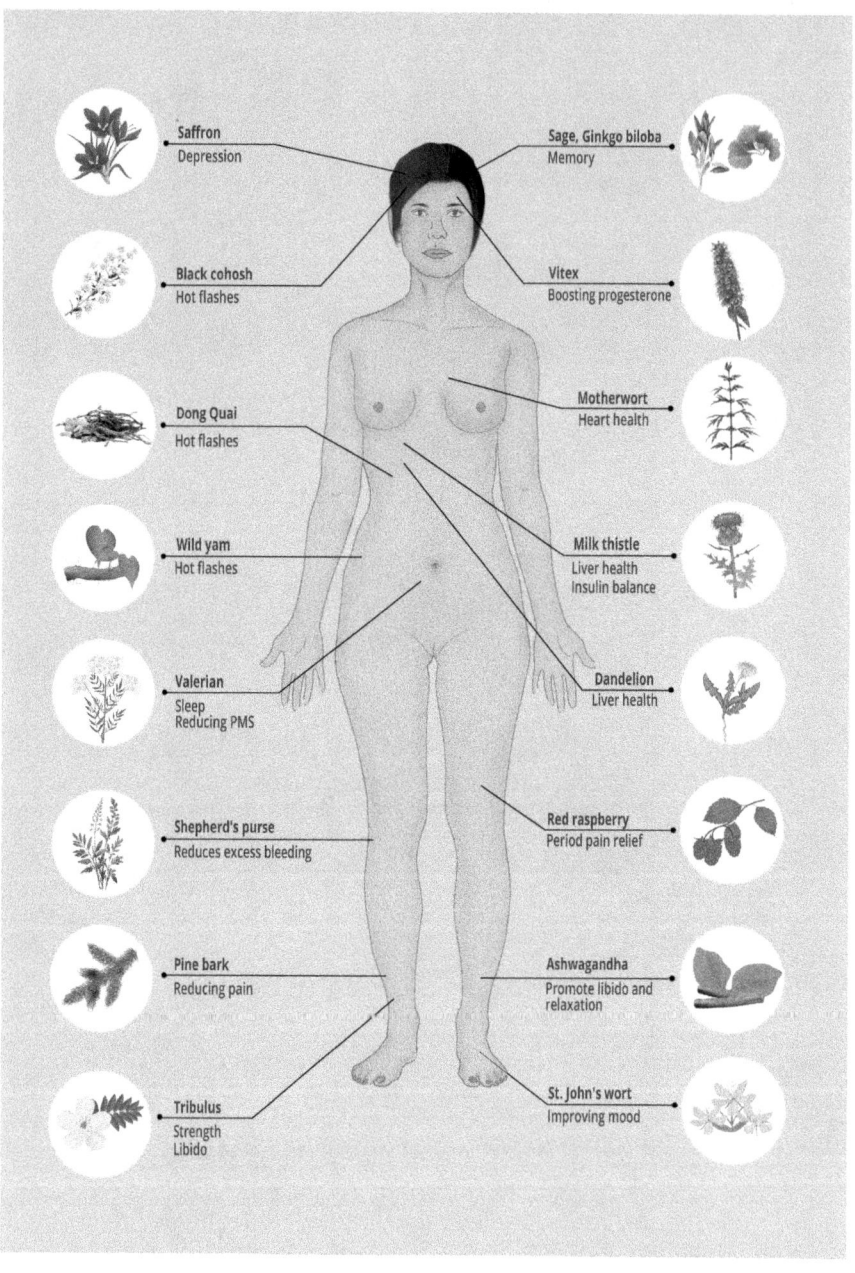

Figure 2: Herbs and how they help improve every aspect of hormonal health.

In this chapter, I will give you a beginner's knowledge of many herbs and their fascinating benefits for the women's reproductive system. This isn't a complete list, but it will help get you started on the path of herbal and natural healing. It will help you have a discussion with your provider about your own best personal health journey. Just so you know, I personally have tried and used all of these herbs either intermittently or daily depending on their function and my health goals.

Then in Chapter 6 and 7, I will explore with you when each natural remedy may be helpful for certain hormonal and women's issues.

Natural Remedies from the Earth

When looking for herbs, there are a couple of important points to keep in mind. Tea forms as well as herbs found in recipes and beverages are safe. The only downside I see to using tea forms and recipes with herbs is that it is often hard to keep your use of these plants consistently. For this reason alone, I find that using capsules and tinctures of herbs is easier and more effective personally.

If you are taking herbs as supplements in capsules or tinctures, look for standardized extracts and companies with third-party testing known as certified Good Manufacturing Practices (cGMP). This will be listed on the label. Additionally, you should try to seek out herbal dispensaries that are reputable such as Fullscript as discussed on page 59. You can also often find good herbal suppliers in your local community through compounding pharmacies and in reputable markets such as Natural Grocers. You should know that some retailers and online marketplaces sell fake products and this is exactly the opposite of what you should buy.

Chapter 5

When it comes to dosing of herbals, there are often unknowns, but this doesn't mean that they should be avoided or discouraged. Rather, the dosing recommendations on supplement labels are very conservative most of the time. For this reason, it helps to stick to the dosing recommendations on the label unless your healthcare provider recommends a different amount. Growing your own herbs is also a great option, and in this case, I recommend using the herbs in tea form, in homemade salves, homemade tinctures, or in culinary recipes.

These are really easy to make too. I will share with you how I make my own salves and tinctures.

Just so we are all on the same page:

- **A tincture** is simply an herbal extract in liquid form
- **A salve** is an oil-based tincture that is thickened by beeswax that can be used topically

My preferred method is an oil-based tincture because it is quick to make and can be more mellow-tasting than alcohol-based tinctures. You can take the herbal tincture straight without mixing it into water because of this.

One downside to making your own tinctures is that you can't know exactly how much herb you are getting. But don't let this deter you from trying your hand at making your own because it can be very rewarding and less expensive than the ones you purchase. Salves are very effective because the skin absorbs natural compounds without negative side effects. I especially like using salves for localized pain relief. I also love topical wild yam salve and natural hormone creams.

For alcohol-based tincture:

- Fill a jar ½ to ¾ of the way with your chopped flowers, herbs, or roots

- Top it off and cover with alcohol such as vodka
- Strain the alcohol with a cheesecloth after your desired strength is achieved, often 1 week to a month after infusing. If you don't mind the herbal pieces, you can also consume them. Place the newly-made herbal extract in a tincture bottle. You can find these online or in herbal stores.

For oil-based tincture:

- Add your chopped herb of choice to a double boiler and cover it with extra virgin olive oil. Heat it to 150 degrees Fahrenheit using a candy thermometer, using care to not heat the oil to over 175 degrees.
- Allow the mixture to infuse for about an hour or so.
- Strain the oil using a cheese cloth and place the oil in a tincture bottle. You can find these online or in herbal stores.

Sturdier herbs can work best for this method, such as lavender, cannabis, and sage. People who try this method for making tinctures are rarely disappointed because the whole plant is preserved and the oil delivery method makes it absorb more readily into the body.

Note for cannabis tincture: before infusing cannabis into a tincture, you should first activate (decarboxylate) it by baking it at a low temperature, about 225 degrees Fahrenheit for 25-30 minutes. Once it cools down a bit, break it into very small pieces with your hands before adding it to a double boiler in the first step above.

For a homemade salve:
   Simply follow the directions for making an oil tincture. Heat the infused oil in a double boiler at 150 F with organic beeswax. I use a ratio of 2 cups of oil to 1/2 cup of beeswax. Use more or less depending on your desired consistency.

Chapter 5

***

Harnessing Your Women's Health with Herbs

In this section, I encourage you to explore the fascinating herbal benefits for finding your inner sanctum. I suggest starting with the ones that have the most research and then follow these up with ones that have a long history of traditional use but less research behind them. I list them in order of the strength of research that they have.

But keep in mind that just because there isn't research behind some doesn't mean they aren't effective. In my experience, these herbs can be even more effective than those with stacks of research about them. Some of my favorites have traditional uses that stand the test of time without research. After all, no big pharmaceutical companies with a ton of money are going to fund a study about something that will never make them any money because it grows right in your garden.

Might these big companies and even "authoritative" websites discourage you from using herbs because they stand to lose money from a movement towards natural medicine? I'll leave that for you to decide.

Vitex-The All-Purpose Herb

If there was an herb that could do everything but wash the dishes, it is Vitex. Research on this plant's benefits is quite extensive. Of all the hormone-balancing herbs, Vitex is very effective for many women at any age; from your first period to your last one and beyond. This incredible plant reduces premenstrual syndrome symptoms, including breast tenderness, swelling, excess bleeding, bloating, and mood swings.[4] In fact, it works as well as some antidepressant medications for improving mood. It may even help reduce PCOS symptoms and help boost fertility. Vitex is also able to help reduce headaches and migraines associated with PMS[5]. All the while, Vitex is known for helping increase progesterone too, so it can help reduce a heavy period flow. Using Vitex helps minimize the abnormal bleeding that comes from having IUDs (intrauterine devices).[5] Just keep in mind that it may take a few months of using Vitex to achieve optimal effectiveness. A common daily dose is 750-1000 mg per day. Look for brands that contain Vitex standardized to contain 0.5% agnuside which is one of the active anti-inflammatory components of Vitex. And side effects are quite rare, but occasionally can cause some temporary nausea. Take it with food to avoid any nausea. Like anything, if you do have lasting side effects from it, you should not take it.

Saffron-The Uplifting Beauty

This beautiful and healing plant is amazing for mood and helps promote a normal menstrual cycle as reviewed above in the Harmonious Herbs section on page 89. In addition to the benefits for reducing anxiety and depression mentioned previously, saffron may also improve sexual desire and function. It even works to do so in the setting of antidepressant prescription medication-caused sexual dysfunction.[6] Not that this book is about men, but it also helps improve erectile dysfunction[7]. And hey, we definitely want men to be healthy too. The typical dose used is 30 mg per day, which is a very small amount for such powerful effects. I personally love this plant because I definitely notice an improvement in my mood and notice it pretty rapidly. More isn't necessarily better either-low doses are sufficient to have beneficial effects and pregnant women should avoid doses greater than 5000 mg per day.

Chapter 5

Black Cohosh for Low Estrogen Symptoms

Black cohosh is a traditional medicine that is used for easing menstrual cramps, PMS, and for also alleviating menopausal symptoms. This beneficial herb is most likely to help women who are struggling with low estrogen, including women who exercise heavily, restrict their food intake for weight loss, women with anxiety, and women entering into menopause and beyond. Personally, I've tried this herb in the past, and by matter of inclusion, I learned that I wasn't low in estrogen at all, rather, I was low in progesterone. But, as I get closer to menopause, I am finding this herb to be very beneficial now. This is because research shows that black cohosh reduces hot flashes and improves mood according to the Spanish Menopause Society and according to a review of 22 clinical research papers.[8-9]

Research also shows that black cohosh works better than evening primrose oil for alleviating menopausal symptoms.[10] As an antioxidant-rich plant, black cohosh may also reduce joint pain from arthritis. Some people worry that black cohosh may be harmful for people going through breast cancer because it helps reduce menopausal symptoms. Luckily for us, black cohosh is not estrogenic. Rather, this herb is an estrogen agonist and **selective estrogen receptor modulator** (SERM) which means that it may be helpful rather than harmful in estrogenic-type cancers[11]. Two studies to date show that black cohosh use has significant protective effects against breast cancer development because the herb itself has anticancer properties.[11-12]

Try to find black cohosh that is standardized to 2.5% triterpene glycosides. Brands like Nature's Way and Now Brand meet this criteria. Using doses of around 40 mg per day are effective for helping reduce hot flashes.[13]

Ashwagandha for the "Oh Wow"

When I was digging into the research of various plant remedies, one that surprised me in terms of how it helps augment the women's reproductive system is ashwagandha. I knew it helped dampen cortisol, but its striking benefits during the life cycle is very interesting. Also known as winter cherry, Ashwagandha helps improve low estrogen levels and helps reduce **genitourinary symptoms** for women during perimenopause. In other words, it helps sexual function while also reducing the psychological symptoms of menopause. The study that examined these benefits was of the highest quality according to science's standards: a double-blind, placebo-controlled study.[14] I'm pleased to announce that another recent study also found very similar results for improving the sexual function of healthy women of all ages between 18-50 years old, so it's not just for "women of a certain age".[15] The sexual function that the study mentioned is lubrication, orgasm, interest in sex, and total sexual function. Another impressive part of this study is that the results continued to improve over the 8-week period indicating that it was a true result, not the result of a placebo. Generally speaking, ashwagandha is healthy too because it dampens the stress response.[16] It also helps improve immune response and acts as a potent antioxidant in the body. Some research shows it reduces fatigue and this could be because it helps optimize thyroid levels.[17] And yep, you guessed it; Ashwagandha also helps improve memory and focus without any meaningful side effects.[18] Research studies use doses between 250-300 mg per day, but you will commonly find that people supplement around 500-1000 mg per day without any side effects. While some websites caution against its use if you have hormone-sensitive cancers, this is based on speculation and not facts as ashwagandha in and of itself has properties in it that may reduce cancer risk, even reduce breast cancer risk.[19] Used for thousands of years in cultures that have low cancer incidence, there seems little cause for alarm. But if you do have hormone-sensitive cancer risk, make sure to discuss ashwagandha with your healthcare provider.

Tulsi-Liquid Yoga

Tulsi, aka Holy Basil, is a personal favorite of mine to help with stress and adaptation. It is considered sacred in Hinduism and also referred to as liquid yoga. Sometimes I have two cups of tulsi tea daily to support relaxation and focus. This **adaptogen herb** is grown sustainably and is clinically shown in many research studies to reduce stress, the father of backhanded cortisol, with 30-40 percent symptom reduction in stress.[20] You might be surprised to know that early research shows that it is as effective as prescription Valium (diazepam) for stress without all the terrible side effects and addiction of this drug.[21] And even better, it improves memory instead of worsening it like the pharmaceuticals out there for anxiety. If that wasn't enough, this fascinating herb helps reduce diabetes symptoms which, in turn, naturally will help reduce PCOS and other hormonal issues.[22] A review of 14 clinical studies found tulsi beneficial for many aspects of health for people with diabetes, including improved blood pressure, reduced cholesterol levels, and improved blood sugar numbers.[22] Doses of 1200 mg a day have been used for its anxiety-relieving effects. Higher doses seem to work better than lower doses and lucky for us, tulsi is generally regarded as safe.

Milk Thistle-A Powerful Plant

Used primarily to support a healthy liver, milk thistle also is amazing for hormone balancing in PCOS and menopausal and perimenopausal symptoms. One of the reasons people struggle with PCOS or polycystic ovarian syndrome is because their bodies can mount an excessive inflammatory response. Milk thistle is a great remedy for inflammation. Herbal medicines like milk thistle can also help reduce many other symptoms of PCOS. This is because it has beneficial effects on blood glucose levels and its antioxidant effects also help increase fertility rates.[23] Research even shows that herbal medicines like milk thistle help improve hormone levels in people with PCOS symptoms.[24] Also, women going through menopause often struggle with hot flashes and many other symptoms like brain fog, fatigue, and weight gain. Luckily, milk thistle helps reduce hot flashes symptoms and fatigue in women who are struggling with these symptoms.[25] Try to find milk thistle that is standardized to contain 80% silymarin flavonoids. Now brand milk thistle supplement fits the bill and also contains dandelion root which is great for symptoms of PMS. Doses typically range from 70-140 mg three times daily. You can learn all about milk thistle on my blog here: https://thehealthyrd.com/milk-thistle-for-ibs-liver-health-and-more/

Turmeric to the Rescue

As you may recall, too much estrogen is a problem for many women and can lead to abnormal menstrual cycles like excess bleeding and irregular periods. If you have inflammation, as most people living in Westernized countries do, you should know that inflammation causes disruption to ovulation and thyroid function.[26] Some other examples of women's conditions associated with too much inflammation are PCOS, PMS, hormonal acne, **fibroids**, infertility, endometriosis, hot flashes, perimenopause, and menopause. This is where turmeric comes in. A potent anti-inflammatory without the stronger dangers of prescription anti-inflammatory medications, turmeric can help the menstrual cycle in so many ways. It even supports releasing a healthy egg for fertility.[27] Turmeric not only dampens pain due to menstruation, it also gets to the root problem of hormones by supporting liver detoxification of hormones like estrogen.[28] It also helps support normal digestive function and absorption of fats by promoting normal bile flow. These fats that you need to absorb are hormone precursors. But don't expect turmeric to work overnight. Studies show that giving it at least a week before menstruation is critical for dampening period symptoms like PMS and menstrual cramps. Cooking with turmeric is a great option if you plan on using it regularly. For many people adding a turmeric supplement is a smart option to have a consistent amount in the diet. Doses of around 500 mg of turmeric as curcumin supplements are used in studies and I encourage you to find a supplement of it with black pepper, often listed as Bioperine and please also take it with a fatty meal to enhance its absorption. Still, I've noticed that some people don't tolerate turmeric, and if this is you, another option you could try is Boswellia for similar effects.

Valerian Root-Nature's Better-Than Valium

If you aren't familiar with Valerian root, you should be. Classically used as an effective herbal sleep aid, I was surprised to find quite a bit of research about how Valerian Root also helps reduce hormonal symptoms, including menopause and PMS symptoms.[29] As with all medicinal herbs, this plant contains a multitude of healthy compounds including terpenes, flavonoids, and even contains natural GABA, a calming neurotransmitter. Not surprisingly, it also improves sleep quality in women.[33] As a natural **phytoestrogen**, this plant helps balance hormones all the while not having negative risks of synthetic hormone replacement (such as increased cancer risk). If all that wasn't enough, this plant also reduces anxiety and obsessive compulsive disorder symptoms.[34] And this is likely part of how Valerian root helps balance hormones, throughout the lifespan, without the negative side effects of anti-anxiety drugs. Using 530 mg twice daily of this relaxing herb significantly reduces hot flashes in multiple studies.[30-32] It is also effective in doses of 255 mg given 3 times daily. Just be aware that this medicinal plant has a characteristic smell, which isn't super pleasant but if it smells a bit like a foot, you know you got the right stuff.

Red Raspberry Leaf- A Gentle Period Regulator

Technically a food, red raspberry leaf is perhaps the safest, yet most gentle plant out there that can really help you regulate your menstrual cycles. Red raspberry leaf tea has long been used as a hormone-balancing tea and a uterine tonic. According to research, it may help improve labor and delivery.[35] It may also reduce preterm labor and post-term labor risks.[36] Fascinatingly, red raspberry leaf also reduces heavy bleeding, also known as menorrhagia, in women.[37-38] Most commonly used to help facilitate labor and childbirth, red raspberry leaf is also very effective for period regulation. It is known as a uterine tonic because it promotes blood flow to the uterus and research shows that it may even improve pregnancy outcomes and reduce morning sickness.[39] A **preclinical** study shows that red raspberry leaf decreases levels of harmful estrogen and testosterone, all while increasing luteinizing hormone (helps release an egg) and FSH increases (helps ovulation).[40] Many women find that using red raspberry leaf helps ease period pain and regulates their menstrual cycle, even PMS, without any negative side effects. Some reviewers find it much more beneficial than using birth control for this purpose. Luckily for us, red raspberry leaf is among the safest of plants to take for hormonal issues and I suggest taking it in capsule form if you want it consistently in your diet. You can also get red raspberry leaf tea or make your own from your garden. Typical doses are between 600-1000 mg per day.

Tribulus is for Vitality and Vigor

Among the many herbs that have lovingly entered my supplement cabinet, Tribulus is one that makes me feel more myself in the perimenopausal years and I can safely take it based on everything I've read about it. This is because this plant has complex and enhancing effects on the reproductive tract which is why it gets its claim to fame as a sexual stimulant. And it's one of the few things like this that work as well or better for women as it does for men. Tribulus is an herb used to help increase muscle mass and helps improve sexual function in women according to clinical research.[41-44] This is because it has a weak testosterone **agonist** effect meaning that it helps testosterone circulate more effectively.[45] It also helps reduce blood pressure and helps manage blood sugar levels. Some solid research even shows that Tribulus helps improve the structure and function of ovaries and uterus in women with PCOS.[46] All the while, this herb reduces the risk of kidney stones, has **cardioprotective** properties, and may reduce hormonal cancers (although more research is needed).[47] What pharmaceutical can stack up to that? Doses between 450-1000mg per day are typically used in research and in supplement extracts of Tribulus.

***

Did you Know....Pine Bark Helps Tackle Many Kinds of Pain

Used traditionally through the winters to prevent scurvy, pine bark is a fascinating plant remedy that performs in so many ways. I originally fell in love with pine bark when I first learned that it was an effective supplement for helping reduce the pain of varicose veins. It really did help my veins stop aching after using it for several weeks. So it makes sense that pine bark can help with other painful conditions and it does. Scientists know that it helps with are endometriosis, period pain, and sexual function along with perimenopause.[48-50] People with endometriosis taking pine bark had much less need for pain medications when taking 60 mg pine bark per day and the longer women took it, the better it worked for reducing pain. Another study found it works overall well for painful periods but helped more after the second month as it did in the endometriosis study. And like so many other plants, pine bark has side benefits in that it improves sexual function in perimenopausal women all the while improving their cholesterol numbers. I really can't describe how amazing plants can be, including pine bark. The intelligence built within them is humbling and such a gift to our bodies. To ignore these gifts is like denying our bodies breaths of air. What side effects does pine bark have? None. Zero. Zilch. Except, of course, if you are allergic to it. Doses used in studies ranged from 60-200 mg per day.

Maca-The Energy Booster

Maca isn't really an herb at all, but is a cruciferous vegetable that has been used traditionally as medicine in South America for respiratory conditions and as an aphrodisiac. A limited amount of research shows that it is indeed helpful for these purposes. But another benefit for maca has been uncovered: it reduces fatigue in women, which is pretty great[51]. While there is minimal research on this plant for hormones, it carries a benefit of reducing menopausal symptoms according to a review of 4 clinical trials.[52] People typically use 1-3 grams of maca per day, and hey, it's a vegetable so it's pretty safe. But because it is a vegetable related to broccoli, some people can get a little gassy especially when first using this. You should also be aware that this herb can feel stimulating like caffeine and can cause some irritability symptoms. If this is you, decrease the dose or stop taking maca.

Cannabis-The Endocannabinoid Regulator

Did you know that we all have an **endocannabinoid system** and that many foods we eat have natural cannabinoids in them? These foods include most spices, herbs, and even broccoli! The endocannabinoid system regulates much of our mood, how well we sleep, appetite, learning abilities, growth, nerve transmission, and much more.[53] Cannabis just happens to be a concentrated source of cannabinoids called THC and CBD among other cannabinoids that it contains.

Sadly, cannabis is a very polarizing herb in the news and even in research. Bias about this medicinal plant goes way back, but the truth of this herb is that if used properly and with a deep understanding of how it works, it can literally be life-changing for the better for many people. Because it was illegal since the 1970s and then became legal again for many people in the 2000s, it retains a mystique and has shame around it, but it shouldn't be that way. Historically, presidents have grown cannabis as hemp for its amazing durability of a plant. George Washington and James Madison both grew hemp crops! Intentional misinformation, greed, and racism spun some of the recent negative connotations of using this plant and led to its illegal status.[54] But it's important to also remember that it was listed in the US Pharmacopeia and openly sold as medicine dating back to the 1800s in the United States[54].

As an amazing pain reliever, this herb is far superior to many pain relievers in that cannabis doesn't increase the risk of kidney failure like **non-steroidal anti-inflammatory medications** do or death from opiates.[55] And, many women take enough ibuprofen to increase their kidney failure risk due to menstrual pain or endometrial issues. Cannabis isn't without its risks for sure, but the risks are fewer and further between than people think if used as a whole plant like it is supposed to be.

* * *

Did You Know....How to Safely and Effectively Introduce Cannabis

*Topical use of a high-quality cannabis salve can be one of the best routes of delivery of cannabis especially for people who are worried about the **psychoactive** effects of this plant. The quality of edible cannabis and tinctures vary greatly in dispensaries so I highly suggest that you make your own from the cannabis buds instead of buying pre-made edibles (see page 93 for how to make your own tinctures and salves). If you do buy pre-made edibles, make sure that there is CBD in your edibles otherwise you are WAY more likely to have negative side effects. After all, both CBD and THC are naturally found in this healing plant. However, research studies conducted by people who don't understand the plant well end up manipulating the data by using THC only. This isn't good science and isn't good medicine for people who want herbal medicine to be based on herb's ability to have its own natural checks and balances. Cannabis, like all other herbs, has its own checks and balances in it if humans don't get in the way of it. Also, cannabis as the whole flower not only has THC and CBD, which are antioxidants themselves, it contains a multitude of healing compounds. This includes compounds called terpenes and phenols which are great not only for pain but great for the immune system. Cannabis also likely reduces cancer risk and can be healing for neurological conditions.[56]*

Still, research about the effects of cannabis and the women's reproductive system are in their infancy, but from countless experience over thousands of years, this is a great plant for reducing pain and mood swings around period time. I highly recommend that you learn about dosing and how to use cannabis by checking out a podcast called Cannabis Health Radio. It takes time and adaptation to this plant, so you often really have to be invested in trusting in your endocannabinoid system, which can vary from day to day. Because there is some uncertainty about using cannabis in a developing brain, cannabis should be reserved for adult use in most cases. In any study where negative associations are found around cannabis, remember that the data was collected for these studies when it still retained its illegal status, meaning that these studies have a level of bias behind them that is insurmountable. In other words, it's not very believable. One note of caution; while the research is of very poor quality, some early research suggests that cannabis may impair ovulation in the short term but after longer-term use, adaptation to cannabis makes it so that hormones aren't affected by it.[57] Interestingly, several early studies showed that women had very little to no distress about their periods while using cannabis.[58-61] But because we don't really know much about it during pregnancy, it makes sense to limit it or avoid it during pregnancy.

St. John's Wort: 4-in-1 For Mood

If there ever was a case of science following nature, it is St. John's wort. A natural antidepressant, this herb has identical benefits to SSRI medications without as many negative side effects. Remember, plants have their own built-in checks and balances and this is likely why people have less bad effects using the herb over the pharmaceutical. Unlike SSRI medications and most other medications, St. John's wort reduces the **reuptake** of serotonin, dopamine, and norepinephrine, all the while helping reduce stress hormones so it acts like a 4-in-1 for mood.[62-63] While I'm not suggesting that you self-treat depression I do want to point out that nature gets it right most often. In the context of women's hormones and menstrual cycles, St. John's wort helps to reduce hot flashes and reduces physical and behavioral PMS symptoms as well as menopausal symptoms in clinical studies.[64-67] When it is combined with the herb Vitex, it works even better than alone.[68] All the while St. John's wort on its own helps improve women's quality of life and sexual function which is pretty huge.[69-70] It does all of this without altering hormones, so the true mechanism of how it works in these cases is unknown. However, it may work to help metabolize hormones into their less harmful forms. Doses of 100-300 mg three times daily are often used in research. If you are on birth control, you should check with your doctor before taking St. John's wort because it may decrease the circulating levels of the drug.[71]

Ginger-A Warming Spice for Pain Relief

I bet no one so far has shared with you that a review of 7 clinical trials examined the use of ginger for abnormal periods, but it's true.[72] In fact, ginger root works well for painful periods if given a few days before and during the menstrual period.[73-74] In these studies, the doses of ginger ranged from 750-2000 mg of ginger, usually split up into doses of 250-500 mg three times daily.[75] They used it effectively in women who have severe pain who respond poorly to the use of standard medications like ibuprofen.[76] Not surprisingly, people in the placebo group withdrew because they couldn't handle the pain, while the ginger group had symptom relief similar to the relief that ibuprofen studies have shown. Some research even shows that ginger root supplementation over a 3-month period reduces menstrual blood loss.[77] And unlike over-the-counter pain relievers, ginger is rich in antioxidants that dampen inflammation and even reduces the risk of cancer. As a bonus, most people's digestive tracts benefit from extra ginger due to its warming effects and how it enhances gut muscle movements. When combined with frankincense, ginger reduces menstrual bleeding significantly and improves quality of life better than ibuprofen.

Shepherd's Purse to Slow the Flow

Shepherd's purse is a plant in the broccoli family that is used to reduce bleeding and that it does according to traditional medicine and some clinical research. It got its name from the fact that shepherds would carry it with them on their voyages to reduce bleeding from wounds. Research shows that it does reduce bleeding; one study found that Shepherd's Purse reduced bleeding after birth better than the hormone called oxytocin.[78] Using 500 mg of Shepherd's Purse every 12 hours reduced menstrual bleeding better than an anti-inflammatory drug called mefenamic acid.[79]

As a member of the broccoli family it is rich in some of the same anti-cancer and compounds that detoxify estrogen as well. Beyond that, Shepherd's purse is anti-inflammatory and has strong antibacterial effects.[80] Some people experience some drowsiness when using Shepherd's purse, but you know what makes people even more drowsy? Bleeding too much from menstruation. No upper level of intake has been established and no toxicity data has been established because this plant hasn't gotten the attention it deserves. However, no case reports of issues have been reported with this plant. Herbalists usually recommend that you take this herb only during menstruation when you want to slow the flow. My naturopath suggested that I take it every month at the first onset of bleeding and it works very well if I do this. If I wait until bleeding has commenced for a while it seems to be less effective. If you are on blood thinners, this herb is one you should skip.

Sage-Delicious and Powerful

I love making sage tea because it grows like a weed in my garden and I find that it is very calming and focusing. But it does a lot more for women than chilling us out. Over 900 types of sage are available, all with slightly different characteristics but most research focuses on common sage, clary sage, and Spanish sage varieties. Classically used to improve memory as its name would imply, sage has so many other health benefits for people as well. Sage benefits the body because it has antioxidant properties, meaning it can potentially help shut down excessive inflammation, which is a root cause of so many period issues.[80] Sage also has compounds that may inhibit cancer growth.[81] Also, sage activates **PPARγ** which is a regulator of genes involved in energy as well as fat and glucose metabolism. This herb reduces inflammation and has clinically been studied to improve memory and it does so by protecting nerve factors. Luckily for us, sage also benefits hormonal symptoms for women. A variety of sage called clary sage is beneficial for pain because it contains substances like β-caryophyllene. Sage also helps decrease cortisol, which in turn likely helps balance out all the sex hormones. Inhaling sage essential oil reduces cortisol levels in menopausal women.[82] It also has anti-depressant effects and may dampen anxiety. Traditional uses of sage are many and include the ability to alleviate menopausal symptoms in women. One study indeed showed that sage reduces menopause symptoms including hot flashes after 8 weeks of use. Further, hot flashes continued to be reduced with each week of use and provided maximal reduction at 8 weeks of use.[83] No significant side effects of using sage for menopausal symptoms were reported in this study. A common dose of sage supplements is 1000 mg per day, although research hasn't fully vetted out the multitude of doses available and how often to use it. Tinctures are also a popular way to use sage for hormonal symptoms.

Black Cumin Seed-A Master for All Seasons and Reasons

This culinary spice has long been used as an Aruvedic medicine because it effectively reduces symptoms of pain. Black cumin seed is related to the buttercup plant and is a beauty that tastes amazing and a little bit spicy. But like many other herbs and spices, this plant does so much more. Using black cumin seed oil has the ability to help lower blood sugar. This is part of why it helps people with their weight loss efforts and helps with PCOS. This tasty seed is great at reducing glucose absorption and improving glucose tolerance by enhancing insulin sensitivity. For these reasons, black seed oil may help people who have Type 2 Diabetes.[84] Black seed oil helps lower blood sugar and may do so by increasing **insulin receptor** production and reducing inflammation.[90] Research suggests black seed oil reduces fasting glucose levels by almost 30% compared to standard treatment which reduces fasting glucose by 18 percent.[91] Several other studies have confirmed the beneficial effects of black seed oil on diabetes symptoms as well.[92] Anything that helps manage blood sugar and glucose control also helps with sex hormones and thyroid hormones. And, research confirms that black cumin seed indeed helps thyroid function and helps restore estrogen levels in postmenopausal women.[93-94]

This plant is a favorite of mine to incorporate into my daily anti-inflammatory diet. A common dose is 1000 mg per day and I personally use Now Brand Black Cumin Seed Oil. I have noticed a big variability in effectiveness between brands of black cumin seed, so be aware that if you try one brand and it doesn't help, give another brand a try or use ground black cumin seeds. I haven't noticed that it really affects my menstrual cycles per se, but I love its benefits for my joints. But this could be because I carefully regulate my diet anyway on most days, use lots of herbs, and don't suffer from glucose issues.

Cinnamon-A Tasty Spice That Performs

While cinnamon is used commonly to add a nice flavor to foods, few people know about its ability to help with women's menstrual pain and may reduce bleeding amounts. It even has been clinically shown in a pool of 5 studies to reduce the symptoms of PCOS because of its great ability to help regulate blood sugar.[95] Adding to the growing evidence that cinnamon improves hormones is a compilation study of 11 studies showing that cinnamon helps reduce insulin resistance and improves fasting glucose levels.[96] For menstrual cramps, doses of 420 mg 3 times daily are used during the menstrual flow.[97] Make sure to find true cinnamon supplements which are also called Ceylon cinnamon. This is because many cinnamon supplements use the cheaper forms of cinnamon that are more likely to cause side effects.

Period Fix

* * *

Did You Know…Wild Yam and Deception in Media

If there ever was an example of how the spread of health information is quite ridiculous, it is in the area of herbs and particularly wild yam. Every major health website cautions that there are no clinical research studies supporting the use of wild yam, which happens to be true if you look at surface level. However, wild yam is a great source of a compound called diosgenin which is a precursor to all sex hormones and even corticosteroids which regulate inflammation and mineral balance in the body. The diosgenin compound from wild yams has a substantial amount of preclinical research related to its potential to reduce the risk and help alleviate all sorts of neurological conditions, help improve mood, protect against Alzheimer's disease, cancer, and more.[98] It has anti-inflammatory as well as antioxidant effects that may reduce diabetes symptoms and thus help manage hormonal balance in the body.[98] Many women use wild yam topically, including myself. If nothing else, it's great for the skin, but I'm sure it does much more than that based on historical uses for women's health. Many people find it exceptionally beneficial for reducing excess periods and it has massive potential to reduce neurological conditions and more. Did you know that industry makes natural progesterone from wild yam as well as a lot of types of commercial prescriptions?[99] If you trust the internet, which I don't always, it says that diosgenin can't be converted into progesterone in the body. But this claim that it doesn't convert to progesterone has no science to support it. Talk about a double standard!

I'm not saying this means wild yam has all the same biological activities as these prescriptions (thank goodness). When a compound, such as wild yam, is upstream in metabolic processes, often is safer and better than a downstream drug. The only potential downside that I can find of using oral wild yam supplements is that it contains a lot of oxalates if not prepared correctly. For people who have kidney issues related to oxalates, I suggest avoiding using oral wild yam supplements.[100-101] *The workaround is to use it topically which I suggest. The bottom line is that most women who use wild yam cream love it for helping regulate their cycles. Currently, the most highly-rated wild yam cream is from a company called Indian Meadow Herbals Wild Yam Root Cream. Many women find that this cream cures or greatly alleviates their hot flashes, perimenopausal, and postmenopausal symptoms.*

* * *

Ginkgo-A Wise Way to Improve Memory and the Menopause Years

Ginkgo biloba trees are known as a living fossil because, unlike all other trees, it has no known plant relatives and because it lived as far back as the Jurassic period in time. Traditionally the seeds of Ginkgo were considered the medicinal part of the plant but now the leaves are used as well. The leaves alone contain a mixture of around 300 active components. In research, the leaves of this plant have been successful in helping people control diabetes, high blood pressure, and obesity. Ginkgo also has the amazing ability to reduce estrogen by increasing its metabolism into less harmful forms.[102-103] By doing these things, you can imagine that they also support healthy fertility and help manage PCOS. Acting as a **phytoestrogen**, some research suggests that ginkgo is a great alternative to hormone replacement therapy for these reasons. Human studies of this age-old plant demonstrate that it is helpful for reducing PMS symptoms.[104-105] Another great benefit of ginkgo is that it improves memory in the 4 most recent research studies although earlier studies were mixed on this topic likely to do with lower dosages being used.[106-107] Typical doses effectively used in research are around 120-240 mg of Ginkgo per day. People who try Ginkgo are often surprised that it works better than they anticipate for memory and well-being and this supplement has little to no expected side effects.

Nettles-Impressive Overall Tonic

Eaten as a vegetable in some countries, nettles are sadly misunderstood and underused in Western cultures. Many people are surprised when I tell them that nettles supplements are one that I won't live without especially when I get seasonal allergies. But this is because nettles work as well or better than common over-the-counter antihistamines for many people without any of the negative side effects that these drugs bring.[108] For women around the time of their periods, nettles help because it has a natural **diuretic** effect which can ease symptoms of bloating and discomfort and early research shows it helps reduce pain generally. Its rich antioxidant and anti-inflammatory effects also help reduce joint pain and reduce the risk of urinary tract infections. Like many other plants listed here, nettles also reduce hot flashes effectively.[109] One study even found that using topical nettles cream helped improve menopause by reducing vaginal atrophy and vaginal dryness.[110] Traditional use of nettles also suggests that this herb can help with reducing excess menstrual bleeding. All-in-all this nutritious plant doesn't sting at all when you supplement it; it calms down a lot of unpleasant symptoms that make periods worse. And not that this book is about men, but you should also know that nettles help reduce the chances of prostate issues. You can drink nettles tea several times daily. Nettles supplements are very safe and you can take 4000-6000 mg daily.

Chapter 5

Dong Quai- Women's Ginseng

Dong Quai is a time-honored herb in the carrot and celery family that has been long used as a part of traditional Chinese medicine to relieve pain, improve immune function, improve circulation, and to help with PMS, menstrual cramps, and menopausal symptoms. Not only used in China, this revered herb has been used for thousands of years for similar purposes in **Ayurvedic** medicine and Arabic medicine. Its active compounds likely reduce heart rhythm abnormalities, reduce excess clotting, and reduce free radicals in the body. While official studies in people are scarce, the ones we do have show that Dong Quai does indeed reduce menopausal symptoms, including hot flashes, and reduces insomnia and fatigue.[111-113] Some research has even been done alongside cancer treatment to help alleviate the side effects of chemotherapy and radiation, but this research, as one might expect, is still considered preliminary. One note of caution: this herb may help reduce the risk of some kinds of cancer, but shouldn't be taken during pregnancy or breast cancer treatment because it is unknown in this area.[114-115] It also makes sense to avoid taking Dong Quai if you are taking other blood-thinning medications. Many women use Dong Quai in herbal blends as is recommended in traditional Chinese medicine. Although no dosing is established for each condition, a typical amount you will see in herbal blends is between 100-1000 mg per day with the higher doses being effective for reducing menstrual pain, improving sleep, reducing menopausal symptoms, and reducing bleeding. With thousands of reviews reporting these benefits, there is a good chance it can help many people. You should know that this herb smells a lot like celery.

Motherwort-the Lionhearted Herb

Motherwort's botanical name is *Leonurus cardiaca* which may give you a clue regarding its benefits for the heart. This herb in the mint family has at least 29 active compounds, and 17 of these have actions that can help treat the underlying issues with menstrual disorders. Because it is in the mint family it is also used in stews, soups, teas, and even for flavoring beer.[116]

Historically used for uterine tonic benefits, this herb has different effects than other herbs in that it may help support regular menstrual cycles in women who have infrequent cycles. It is also clinically beneficial for reducing postpartum bleeding and helping the uterus return to normal after childbirth.[117] One research study even shows that motherwort is indeed good for the heart because it helps reduce anxiety, reduces blood pressure, and is very well tolerated.[118] For these same reasons, it is most certainly good for hormonal health in some women.[119] Beyond that, there aren't any clinical trials on motherwort, but based on its use in foods and historically, it appears pretty safe for most people. Plenty of preclinical studies find that this herb has strong cardioprotective and anti-anxiety components that make this a great herb for women in many cases.[120] However, there is some concern that its use in women who have heavy periods already could make them bleed even more. I take it regularly and don't find that it makes bleeding better or worse, but do find it relaxing. I do notice that the bleeding has much less clotting in it, interestingly. Again, this is just me. Because it is thought to stimulate uterine contractions, this herb shouldn't be taken during pregnancy. Also, because it has blood-thinning potential, it shouldn't be used if you take blood-thinning medications.[121]

Passion Flower for Chill Moods

Passionflower tea is made from a beautiful purple flower that has long been used for nervous conditions like anxiety, insomnia, PMS, and irritability. Now research is showing its benefits for dampening stress and even easing menopausal symptoms equal to that of St. John's Wort.[122-123] Another study found that passionflower decreases stress when used as an add-on treatment to conventional antidepressant medications and as you know, decreasing stress improves hormonal health.[124] Additionally, passionflower may help increase your total amount of sleep time as well.[125] Passionflower is very safe but should be avoided if you are pregnant and should be avoided if you are taking sedative medications. However, most people can help reduce the tension of the day by sipping on a warm cup of passionflower tea.

Dandelion Root: Natural Diuretic

Eating dandelion plants was recorded by the ancient Romans and used as traditional medicine by Arabian doctors among others. Yet scientific experiments have spent little energy trying to figure this plant out. And they rarely differentiate the use of the leaves versus the root, but most herbal formulations as tonics use the root form of this plant. Some research in animals indicates that dandelions have the ability to modulate estrogen receptors. Additionally, dandelions may improve insulin sensitivity and may increase the amount of estrogen and progesterone production in people who have infertility issues, but research is very preliminary in this area.[126-127] One very small clinical study was conducted and found that it is indeed a **diuretic**, proving out its use as traditional medicine.[128] Like all medicinal plants, dandelion is rich in antioxidants like terpenes that dampen down inflammation in the body.[129] It also has components in it that help protect the liver from toxins like acetaminophen.[130]

These are all good things, but you can get too much of a good thing. According to the British Herbal Pharmacopoeia, here are dosing guidelines for dandelion:[131]

- Fresh leaves 4-10 g daily
- Dried leaves 4-10 g daily
- 2-5 ml of leaf tincture, three times a day
- Fresh leaf juice, 1 teaspoon twice daily,
- Fluid extract 1-2 teaspoon daily

- Fresh roots 2-8 g daily
- Dried powder extract 250-1000 mg four times a day

* * *

Damiana- A Witchy and Mysterious Herb

*I remember the first time I heard of the herb Damiana in a dusty herbal book in the library. I was in my twenties and there was absolutely no research available about it. But it seemed witchy and cool because it was supposed to be an aphrodisiac for women and support women as an overall tonic. I was intrigued! Used for over 2000 years as medicine for numerous ailments in the southern part of the United States, Mexico, South and Central America, this herb has some fascinating history. But back then, because there were no clinical trials available, I was too scared to try it. 30 years later, I've finally given this herb a try and find it very calming and a mellow type of tea to have on any day. It tastes very pleasant and mild as a tea. Sadly, 30 years later there is STILL no clinical research but there is definitely some **preclinical** research on this time-honored herb[129]. It has immune-enhancing and antioxidant effects and is considered an **adaptogen** to stress because it contains the relaxing antioxidant called apigenin, which is very helpful for sleep and anxiety.[130-131] It may even enhance sexual function because it promotes healthy **nitric oxide** production. While this herb does have some estrogenic activity, it interestingly has some anti-cancer effects on breast cancer cells according to several early research studies.[131-132] One could argue that there really isn't enough research yet to give this herb a try, but with a track record of 2000 years with absolutely no horrible side effects found, most women should feel safe in trying this herb. Remember, research these days is almost exclusively driven by*

Big Pharma money, so the field is absolutely a minefield of bias and greed. I understand if you are scared to try it because I was at one point too. But, if you are adventurous, this herb so far seems very safe and has some cool relaxing and health-promoting effects. My friend and I have a cup of Damiana tea every lunch hour to help chill out the afternoons at work.

To be more sure about damiana, you can check out Memorial Sloan Kettering Cancer Center's review of damiana's research here: https://www.mskcc.org/cancer-care/integrative-medicine/herbs/damiana

Herbal Blends

The types and arrays of herbs that I have given you so far can seem daunting: how is the best way to piece it all together? It is a good thing that some reputable supplement companies put together blends of herbs and plant therapies that make it so that you need to buy just a couple and not ten of the above. But, I still encourage you to look at the doses and formulations of these herbal blends because they often have less of each active ingredient than you would get if you buy them separately. For instance, Vitanica's Women's Phase I contains Vitex, but not enough for me as I entered perimenopause, so I take Women's Phase I along with Vitex from Vital Nutrients. I also add in tribulus, wild yam cream, progesterone cream, and red raspberry leaf regularly and have added ashwagandha too. And I've never had any negative side effects; only positive side benefits because these plants are amazing for my body.

Here are some herbal blends that I trust and like by reputable brands:

- **Solaray Stages**-they make PMS & Menstrual, Perimenopause, and

Libido blends that I love and think most women will love. Just be aware that some have maca and this is too stimulating for some women.

- **Vitanica Women's Phase I** for PMS and perimenopause.
- **Mary Ruth's Organics Wellness Liquid Drops**-supports overall healthy menstruation.
- **Thorne SAT**- contains milk thistle (as silymarin), turmeric, and artichoke to help with healthy hormone levels, pain reduction, hot flashes, PMS, PCOS, and liver health.
- **Vital Nutrients PMS Support**-contains passion flower, Vitex, Dong Quai, vitamin B6, and Bupleurum falcatum (good for liver health). I suggest taking this with other B-vitamins to promote a balance of B-vitamins in the body.
- **Vital Nutrients Menopause Support**-has Black Cohosh, Dong Quai, Ginkgo, Wild Yam, Sage, a very small amount of Licorice root, and Rehmanniae Extract (supportive for nerve health and immunity).
- **Estrosense**-available-on Natural Factors website, Instacart and Iherb,this supplement has broccoli extracts (calcium D-glucarate, indole-3-carbinol, di-indolylmethane), decaffeinated green tea extract, milk thistle extract, rosemary extract, turmeric extract, and lycopene from tomatoes.
- **Brain MD Happy Saffron Plus**-has a period-soothing and mood-boosting blend of zinc, saffron, and turmeric.

Chapter 5 References

1. Livdans-Forret AB, Harvey PJ, Larkin-Thier SM. Menorrhagia: a synopsis of management focusing on herbal and nutritional supplements, and chiropractic. J Can Chiropr Assoc. 2007 Dec;51(4):235-46. https://www.ncbi.nlm.nih.gov/pmc/articles/PMC2077876/
2. Jackson PA, Forster J, Khan J, Pouchieu C, Dubreuil S, Gaudout D,

Moras B, Pourtau L, Joffre F, Vaysse C, Bertrand K, Abrous H, Vauzour D, Brossaud J, Corcuff JB, Capuron L, Kennedy DO. Effects of Saffron Extract Supplementation on Mood, Well-Being, and Response to a Psychosocial Stressor in Healthy Adults: A Randomized, Double-Blind, Parallel Group, Clinical Trial. Front Nutr. 2021 Feb 1;7:606124. https://www.ncbi.nlm.nih.gov/pmc/articles/PMC7882499/
3. Hausenblas HA, Saha D, Dubyak PJ, Anton SD. Saffron (Crocus sativus L.) and major depressive disorder: a meta-analysis of randomized clinical trials. J Integr Med. 2013 Nov;11(6):377-83. https://pubmed.ncbi.nlm.nih.gov/24299602/
4. van Die MD, Burger HG, Teede HJ, Bone KM. Vitex agnus-castus extracts for women's reproductive disorders: a systematic review of clinical trials. Planta Med. 2013 May;79(7):562-75. https://pubmed.ncbi.nlm.nih.gov/23136064/
5. Yavarikia P, Shahnazi M, Hadavand Mirzaie S, Javadzadeh Y, Lutfi R. Comparing the effect of mefenamic Acid and vitex agnus on intrauterine device induced bleeding. J Caring Sci. 2013 Aug 31;2(3):245-54. https://www.ncbi.nlm.nih.gov/pmc/articles/PMC4134154/
6. Kashani L, Raisi F, Saroukhani S, Sohrabi H, Modabbernia A, Nasehi AA, Jamshidi A, Ashrafi M, Mansouri P, Ghaeli P, Akhondzadeh S. Saffron for treatment of fluoxetine-induced sexual dysfunction in women: randomized double-blind placebo-controlled study. Hum Psychopharmacol. 2013 Jan;28(1):54-60. https://pubmed.ncbi.nlm.nih.gov/23280545/
7. Kashani L, Raisi F, Saroukhani S, Sohrabi H, Modabbernia A, Nasehi AA, Jamshidi A, Ashrafi M, Mansouri P, Ghaeli P, Akhondzadeh S. Saffron for treatment of fluoxetine-induced sexual dysfunction in women: randomized double-blind placebo-controlled study. Hum Psychopharmacol. 2013 Jan;28(1):54-60. https://pubmed.ncbi.nlm.nih.gov/23280545/
8. Castelo-Branco C, Navarro C, Beltrán E, Losa F, Camacho M; on the behalf of the Natural Products Study Group of the Spanish Menopause

Society. Black cohosh efficacy and safety for menopausal symptoms. The Spanish Menopause Society statement. Gynecol Endocrinol. 2022 May;38(5):379-384. https://pubmed.ncbi.nlm.nih.gov/35403534/

9. Sadahiro R, Matsuoka LN, Zeng BS, Chen KH, Zeng BY, Wang HY, Chu CS, Stubbs B, Su KP, Tu YK, Wu YC, Lin PY, Chen TY, Chen YW, Suen MW, Hopwood M, Yang WC, Sun CK, Cheng YS, Shiue YL, Hung CM, Matsuoka YJ, Tseng PT. Black cohosh extracts in women with menopausal symptoms: an updated pairwise meta-analysis. Menopause. 2023 Jul 1;30(7):766-773. https://pubmed.ncbi.nlm.nih.gov/37192826/

10. Mehrpooya M, Rabiee S, Larki-Harchegani A, Fallahian AM, Moradi A, Ataei S, Javad MT. A comparative study on the effect of "black cohosh" and "evening primrose oil" on menopausal hot flashes. J Educ Health Promot. 2018 Mar 1;7:36. https://pubmed.ncbi.nlm.nih.gov/29619387/

11. Fritz H, Seely D, McGowan J, Skidmore B, Fernandes R, Kennedy DA, Cooley K, Wong R, Sagar S, Balneaves LG, Fergusson D. Black cohosh and breast cancer: a systematic review. Integr Cancer Ther. 2014 Jan;13(1):12-29. https://pubmed.ncbi.nlm.nih.gov/23439657/

12. Crone M, Hallman K, Lloyd V, Szmyd M, Badamo B, Morse M, Dinda S. The antiestrogenic effects of black cohosh on BRCA1 and steroid receptors in breast cancer cells. Breast Cancer (Dove Med Press). 2019 Feb 19;11:99-110. https://pubmed.ncbi.nlm.nih.gov/30858726/

13. Mohapatra, S.; Iqubal, A.; Ansari, M.J.; Jan, B.; Zahiruddin, S.; Mirza, M.A.; Ahmad, S.; Iqbal, Z. Benefits of Black Cohosh (*Cimicifuga racemosa*) for Women Health: An Up-Close and In-Depth Review. *Pharmaceuticals* 2022, 15, 278 https://www.mdpi.com/1424-8247/15/3/278

14. Gopal S, Ajgaonkar A, Kanchi P, Kaundinya A, Thakare V, Chauhan S, Langade D. Effect of an ashwagandha (Withania Somnifera) root extract on climacteric symptoms in women during perimenopause: A randomized, double-blind, placebo-controlled study. J Obstet Gynaecol Res. 2021 Dec;47(12):4414-4425. https://pubmed.ncbi.nlm.

nih.gov/34553463/

15. Ajgaonkar A, Jain M, Debnath K. Efficacy and Safety of Ashwagandha (Withania somnifera) Root Extract for Improvement of Sexual Health in Healthy Women: A Prospective, Randomized, Placebo-Controlled Study. Cureus. 2022 Oct 28;14(10):e30787. https://www.ncbi.nlm.nih.gov/pmc/articles/PMC9701317/

16. Lopresti AL, Smith SJ, Malvi H, Kodgule R. An investigation into the stress-relieving and pharmacological actions of an ashwagandha (Withania somnifera) extract: A randomized, double-blind, placebo-controlled study. Medicine (Baltimore). 2019 Sep;98(37):e17186. https://pubmed.ncbi.nlm.nih.gov/31517876/

17. Abdel-Wahhab KG, Mourad HH, Mannaa FA, Morsy FA, Hassan LK, Taher RF. Role of ashwagandha methanolic extract in the regulation of thyroid profile in hypothyroidism modeled rats. Mol Biol Rep. 2019 Aug;46(4):3637-3649. https://pubmed.ncbi.nlm.nih.gov/31203475/

18. Gopukumar K, Thanawala S, Somepalli V, Rao TSS, Thamatam VB, Chauhan S. Efficacy and Safety of Ashwagandha Root Extract on Cognitive Functions in Healthy, Stressed Adults: A Randomized, Double-Blind, Placebo-Controlled Study. Evid Based Complement Alternat Med. 2021 Nov 30;2021:8254344. https://pubmed.ncbi.nlm.nih.gov/34858513/

19. Vashi R, Patel BM, Goyal RK. Keeping abreast about ashwagandha in breast cancer. J Ethnopharmacol. 2021 Apr 6;269:113759. https://pubmed.ncbi.nlm.nih.gov/33359916/\

20. Cohen MM. Tulsi - Ocimum sanctum: A herb for all reasons. J Ayurveda Integr Med. 2014 Oct-Dec;5(4):251-9. https://www.ncbi.nlm.nih.gov/pmc/articles/PMC4296439/

21. Pemminati S, Gopalakrishna HN, Venkatesh V, Rai A, Shetty S, Vinod A, et al. Anxiolytic effect of acute administration of ursolic acid in rats. *Res J Pharm Biol Chem Sci.* 2011;2:431–7. https://japsonline.com/abstract.php?article_id=37&sts=2

22. Jamshidi N, Cohen MM. The Clinical Efficacy and Safety of Tulsi in Humans: A Systematic Review of the Literature. Evid Based

Complement Alternat Med. 2017;2017:9217567. https://www.ncbi.nlm.nih.gov/pmc/articles/PMC5376420/

23. Zarif-Yeganeh M, Rastegarpanah M. Clinical Role of Silymarin in Oxidative Stress and Infertility: A Short Review for Pharmacy Practitioners. J Res Pharm Pract. 2019 Dec 27;8(4):181-188. https://www.ncbi.nlm.nih.gov/pmc/articles/PMC6952757/

24. Ashkar, Fatemeh, Rezaei, Shahla, Salahshoornezhad, Sara, Vahid, Farhad, Gholamalizadeh, Maryam, Dahka, Samaneh Mirzaei and Doaei, Saeid. "The Role of medicinal herbs in treatment of insulin resistance in patients with Polycystic Ovary Syndrome: A literature review" *Biomolecular Concepts*, vol. 11, no. 1, 2019, pp. 57-75. https://www.degruyter.com/document/doi/10.1515/bmc-2020-0005/html?lang=en

25. Saberi Z, Gorji N, Memariani Z, Moeini R, Shirafkan H, Amiri M. Evaluation of the effect of Silybum marianum extract on menopausal symptoms: A randomized, double-blind placebo-controlled trial. Phytother Res. 2020 Dec;34(12):3359-3366. https://pubmed.ncbi.nlm.nih.gov/32762030/

26. Boots CE, Jungheim ES. Inflammation and Human Ovarian Follicular Dynamics. Semin Reprod Med. 2015 Jul;33(4):270-5. https://www.ncbi.nlm.nih.gov/pmc/articles/PMC4772716/

27. Bahrami A, Zarban A, Rezapour H, Agha Amini Fashami A, Ferns GA. Effects of curcumin on menstrual pattern, premenstrual syndrome, and dysmenorrhea: A triple-blind, placebo-controlled clinical trial. Phytother Res. 2021 Dec;35(12):6954-6962. https://pubmed.ncbi.nlm.nih.gov/34708460/

28. Kamal DAM, Salamt N, Yusuf ANM, Kashim MIAM, Mokhtar MH. Potential Health Benefits of Curcumin on women's Reproductive Disorders: A Review. Nutrients. 2021 Sep 7;13(9):3126. https://www.ncbi.nlm.nih.gov/pmc/articles/PMC8471428/

29. Behboodi Moghadam Z, Rezaei E, Shirood Gholami R, Kheirkhah M, Haghani H. The effect of Valerian root extract on the severity of pre menstrual syndrome symptoms. J Tradit Complement Med. 2016 Jan

19;6(3):309-15. https://pubmed.ncbi.nlm.nih.gov/27419099/
30. Jenabi E, Shobeiri F, Hazavehei SMM, Roshanaei G. The effect of Valerian on the severity and frequency of hot flashes: A triple-blind randomized clinical trial. Women Health. 2018 Mar;58(3):297-304. https://pubmed.ncbi.nlm.nih.gov/28278010/#
31. Jenabi E, Khazaei S, Aghababaei S, Moradkhani S. Effect of Fennel-Valerian Extract on Hot Flashes and Sleep Disorders in Postmenopausal Women: A Randomized Trial. J Menopausal Med. 2023 Apr;29(1):21-2. https://pubmed.ncbi.nlm.nih.gov/37160299/
32. Mirabi P, Mojab F. The effects of valerian root on hot flashes in menopausal women. Iran J Pharm Res. 2013 Winter;12(1):217-22. https://ncbi.nlm.nih.gov/pmc/articles/PMC3813196/
33. Bent S, Padula A, Moore D, Patterson M, Mehling W. Valerian for sleep: a systematic review and meta-analysis. Am J Med. 2006 Dec;119(12):1005-12.https://pubmed.ncbi.nlm.nih.gov/17145239/
34. Pakseresht S, Boostani H, Sayyah M. Extract of valerian root (Valeriana officinalis L.) vs. placebo in treatment of obsessive-compulsive disorder: a randomized double-blind study. J Complement Integr Med. 2011 Oct 11;8:/j/jcim.2011.8.issue-1/1553-3840.1465/1553-38 40.1465.xml. https://pubmed.ncbi.nlm.nih.gov/22718671/
35. Bowman R, Taylor J, Muggleton S, Davis D. Biophysical effects, safety and efficacy of raspberry leaf use in pregnancy: a systematic integrative review. BMC Complement Med Ther. 2021 Feb 9;21(1):56. https://www.ncbi.nlm.nih.gov/pmc/articles/PMC7871383/
36. Bowman R, Taylor J, Muggleton S, Davis D. Biophysical effects, safety and efficacy of raspberry leaf use in pregnancy: a systematic integrative review. BMC Complement Med Ther. 2021 Feb 9;21(1):56. https://www.ncbi.nlm.nih.gov/pmc/articles/PMC7871383/
37. Livdans-Forret AB, Harvey PJ, Larkin-Thier SM. Menorrhagia: a synopsis of management focusing on herbal and nutritional supplements, and chiropractic. J Can Chiropr Assoc. 2007 Dec;51(4):235-46. https://www.ncbi.nlm.nih.gov/pmc/articles/PMC2077876/
38. Hudson, Tori. *Women's Encyclopedia of Natural Medicine: Alterna-*

tive Therapies and Integrative Medicine for Total Health and Wellness. MACMILLAN HEINEMANN, 2007.

39. D. Jill Mallory,Chapter 53 - Postdates Pregnancy. Integrative Medicine (Fourth Edition),Elsevier,2018,Pages 535-541.e1. https://www.sciencedirect.com/topics/medicine-and-dentistry/red-raspberry-leaf#
40. Ferlemi AV, Lamari FN. Berry Leaves: An Alternative Source of Bioactive Natural Products of Nutritional and Medicinal Value. Antioxidants (Basel). 2016 Jun 1;5(2):17. https://www.ncbi.nlm.nih.gov/pmc/articles/PMC4931538/
41. Rogerson S, Riches CJ, Jennings C, Weatherby RP, Meir RA, Marshall-Gradisnik SM. The effect of five weeks of Tribulus terrestris supplementation on muscle strength and body composition during preseason training in elite rugby league players. J Strength Cond Res. 2007 May;21(2):348-53. https://pubmed.ncbi.nlm.nih.gov/17530942/
42. Gama CR, Lasmar R, Gama GF, Abreu CS, Nunes CP, Geller M, Oliveira L, Santos A. Clinical Assessment of Tribulus terrestris Extract in the Treatment of women's Sexual Dysfunction. Clin Med Insights Womens Health. 2014 Dec 22;7:45-50. https://pubmed.ncbi.nlm.nih.gov/25574150/
43. de Souza KZ, Vale FB, Geber S. Efficacy of Tribulus terrestris for the treatment of hypoactive sexual desire disorder in postmenopausal women: a randomized, double-blinded, placebo-controlled trial. Menopause. 2016 Nov;23(11):1252-1256. https://pubmed.ncbi.nlm.nih.gov/27760089/
44. Vale FBC, Zanolla Dias de Souza K, Rezende CR, Geber S. Efficacy of Tribulus Terrestris for the treatment of premenopausal women with hypoactive sexual desire disorder: a randomized double-blinded, placebo-controlled trial. Gynecol Endocrinol. 2018 May;34(5):442-445. https://pubmed.ncbi.nlm.nih.gov/29172782/
45. Ghanbari A, Akhshi N, Nedaei SE, Mollica A, Aneva IY, Qi Y, Liao P, Darakhshan S, Farzaei MH, Xiao J, Echeverría J. Tribulus terrestris and women's reproductive system health: A comprehensive review. Phytomedicine. 2021 Apr;84:153462. https://pubmed.ncbi.nlm.nih.g

ov/33602600/

46. Qureshi A, Naughton DP, Petroczi A. A systematic review on the herbal extract Tribulus terrestris and the roots of its putative aphrodisiac and performance enhancing effect. J Diet Suppl. 2014 Mar;11(1):64-79. https://pubmed.ncbi.nlm.nih.gov/33602600/

47. Tribulus terrestris: Purported Benefits, Side Effects & More. Memorial Sloan Kettering Center. https://www.mskcc.org/cancer-care/integrative-medicine/herbs/tribulus-terrestris

48. Suzuki N, Uebaba K, Kohama T, Moniwa N, Kanayama N, Koike K. French maritime pine bark extract significantly lowers the requirement for analgesic medication in dysmenorrhea: a multicenter, randomized, double-blind, placebo-controlled study. J Reprod Med. 2008 May;53(5):338-46. https://pubmed.ncbi.nlm.nih.gov/18567279/

49. Kohama T, Suzuki N, Ohno S, Inoue M. Analgesic efficacy of French maritime pine bark extract in dysmenorrhea: an open clinical trial. J Reprod Med. 2004 Oct;49(10):828-32. https://pubmed.ncbi.nlm.nih.gov/15568408/

50. Yang HM, Liao MF, Zhu SY, Liao MN, Rohdewald P. A randomised, double-blind, placebo-controlled trial on the effect of Pycnogenol on the climacteric syndrome in peri-menopausal women. Acta Obstet Gynecol Scand. 2007;86(8):978-85. https://pubmed.ncbi.nlm.nih.gov/17653885/

51. Fruzzetti, F., Benelli, E., Fidecicchi, T., & Tonacchera, M. (2020). Clinical and metabolic effects of alpha-lipoic acid associated with two different doses of myo-inositol in women with polycystic ovary syndrome. *International Journal of Endocrinology, 2020*, 1–8. https://ffhdj.com/index.php/ffhd/article/view/912

52. Johnson A, Roberts L, Elkins G. Complementary and Alternative Medicine for Menopause. J Evid Based Integr Med. 2019 Jan-Dec;24:2515690X19829380. https://www.ncbi.nlm.nih.gov/pmc/articles/PMC6419242/

53. Skaper SD, Di Marzo V. Endocannabinoids in nervous system health and disease: the big picture in a nutshell. Philos Trans R Soc Lond B

Biol Sci. 2012 Dec 5;367(1607):3193-200. https://www.ncbi.nlm.nih.gov/pmc/articles/PMC3481537/#
54. Weeding Out the Misconceptions: The True History of Marijuana in America, For The People website. https://www.forthepeople.com/blog/the-true-history-of-marijuana-in-america/
55. Román-Vargas Y, Porras-Arguello JD, Blandón-Naranjo L, Pérez-Pérez LD, Benjumea DM. Evaluation of the Analgesic Effect of High-Cannabidiol-Content Cannabis Extracts in Different Pain Models by Using Polymeric Micelles as Vehicles. Molecules. 2023 May 24;28(11):4299. https://pubmed.ncbi.nlm.nih.gov/37298776/
56. Dariš B, Tancer Verboten M, Knez Ž, Ferk P. Cannabinoids in cancer treatment: Therapeutic potential and legislation. Bosn J Basic Med Sci. 2019 Feb 12;19(1):14-23. https://www.ncbi.nlm.nih.gov/pmc/articles/PMC6387667/
57. Brents LK. Marijuana, the Endocannabinoid System and the women's Reproductive System. Yale J Biol Med. 2016 Jun 27;89(2):175-91. https://pubmed.ncbi.nlm.nih.gov/27354844/
58. Seifalian A, Kenyon J, Khullar V. Dysmenorrhoea: Can Medicinal Cannabis Bring New Hope for a Collective Group of Women Suffering in Pain, Globally? Int J Mol Sci. 2022 Dec 19;23(24):16201. https://www.ncbi.nlm.nih.gov/pmc/articles/PMC9780805/
59. Pařízek, A., Suchopár, J., Laštůvka, Z., Alblová, M., Hill, M., & Dušková, M. (2023). The endocannabinoid system and its relationship to human reproduction. *Physiological Research*. https://doi.org/10.33549/physiolres.935229. https://www.biomed.cas.cz/physiolres/pdf/72/72_S365.pdf
60. Griffin ML, Mendelson JH, Mello NK, Lex BW. Marihuana use across the menstrual cycle. Drug Alcohol Depend. 1986 Oct;18(2):213-24. https://pubmed.ncbi.nlm.nih.gov/3780416/#
61. Seifalian A, Kenyon J, Khullar V. Dysmenorrhoea: Can Medicinal Cannabis Bring New Hope for a Collective Group of Women Suffering in Pain, Globally? Int J Mol Sci. 2022 Dec 19;23(24):16201. https://www.ncbi.nlm.nih.gov/pmc/articles/PMC9780805/

62. Franklin M, Cowen PJ. Researching the antidepressant actions of Hypericum perforatum (St. John's wort) in animals and man. Pharmacopsychiatry. 2001 Jul;34 Suppl 1:S29-37. https://pubmed.ncbi.nlm.nih.gov/11518072/
63. Butterweck V, Korte B, Winterhoff H. Pharmacological and endocrine effects of Hypericum perforatum and hypericin after repeated treatment. Pharmacopsychiatry. 2001 Jul;34 Suppl 1:S2-7. https://pubmed.ncbi.nlm.nih.gov/11518068/
64. Canning S, Waterman M, Orsi N, Ayres J, Simpson N, Dye L. The efficacy of Hypericum perforatum (St John's wort) for the treatment of premenstrual syndrome: a randomized, double-blind, placebo-controlled trial. CNS Drugs. 2010 Mar;24(3):207-25. https://pubmed.ncbi.nlm.nih.gov/20155996/
65. Abdali K, Khajehei M, Tabatabaee HR. Effect of St John's wort on severity, frequency, and duration of hot flashes in premenopausal, perimenopausal and postmenopausal women: a randomized, double-blind, placebo-controlled study. Menopause. 2010 Mar;17(2):326-31. https://pubmed.ncbi.nlm.nih.gov/20216274/
66. Donovan JL, DeVane CL, Lewis JG, Wang JS, Ruan Y, Chavin KD, Markowitz JS. Effects of St John's wort (Hypericum perforatum L.) extract on plasma androgen concentrations in healthy men and women: a pilot study. Phytother Res. 2005 Oct;19(10):901-6. https://pubmed.ncbi.nlm.nih.gov/16261523/
67. Liu YR, Jiang YL, Huang RQ, Yang JY, Xiao BK, Dong JX. Hypericum perforatum L. preparations for menopause: a meta-analysis of efficacy and safety. Climacteric. 2014 Aug;17(4):325-35. https://pubmed.ncbi.nlm.nih.gov/24188229/
68. van Die MD, Bone KM, Burger HG, Reece JE, Teede HJ. Effects of a combination of Hypericum perforatum and Vitex agnus-castus on PMS-like symptoms in late-perimenopausal women: findings from a subpopulation analysis. J Altern Complement Med. 2009 Sep;15(9):1045-8. https://pubmed.ncbi.nlm.nih.gov/19757982/
69. Grube B, Walper A, Wheatley D. St. John's Wort extract: efficacy

for menopausal symptoms of psychological origin. Adv Ther. 1999 Jul-Aug;16(4):177-86. https://pubmed.ncbi.nlm.nih.gov/10623319/
70. Al-Akoum M, Maunsell E, Verreault R, Provencher L, Otis H, Dodin S. Effects of Hypericum perforatum (St. John's wort) on hot flashes and quality of life in perimenopausal women: a randomized pilot trial. Menopause. 2009 Mar-Apr;16(2):307-14. https://pubmed.ncbi.nlm.nih.gov/19194342/
71. Berry-Bibee EN, Kim MJ, Tepper NK, Riley HE, Curtis KM. Co-administration of St. John's wort and hormonal contraceptives: a systematic review. Contraception. 2016 Dec;94(6):668-677. https://pubmed.ncbi.nlm.nih.gov/27444983/
72. Daily JW, Zhang X, Kim DS, Park S. Efficacy of Ginger for Alleviating the Symptoms of Primary Dysmenorrhea: A Systematic Review and Meta-analysis of Randomized Clinical Trials. Pain Med. 2015 Dec;16(12):2243-55. https://pubmed.ncbi.nlm.nih.gov/26177393/
73. Rahnama, P., Montazeri, A., Huseini, H.F. et al. Effect of *Zingiber officinale* R. rhizomes (ginger) on pain relief in primary dysmenorrhea: a placebo randomized trial. *BMC Complement Altern Med* 12, 92 (2012). https://bmccomplementmedtherapies.biomedcentral.com/articles/10.1186/1472-6882-12-92
74. Eshaghian R, Mazaheri M, Ghanadian M, Rouholamin S, Feizi A, Babaeian M. The effect of frankincense (Boswellia serrata, oleoresin) and ginger (Zingiber officinale, rhizoma) on heavy menstrual bleeding: A randomized, placebo-controlled, clinical trial. Complement Ther Med. 2019 Feb;42:42-47. https://pubmed.ncbi.nlm.nih.gov/30670277/
75. Daily JW, Zhang X, Kim DS, Park S. Efficacy of Ginger for Alleviating the Symptoms of Primary Dysmenorrhea: A Systematic Review and Meta-analysis of Randomized Clinical Trials. Pain Med. 2015 Dec;16(12):2243-55. https://pubmed.ncbi.nlm.nih.gov/26177393/
76. Shirvani MA, Motahari-Tabari N, Alipour A. The effect of mefenamic acid and ginger on pain relief in primary dysmenorrhea: a randomized clinical trial. Arch Gynecol Obstet. 2015 Jun;291(6):1277-81. https://p

ubmed.ncbi.nlm.nih.gov/25399316/
77. Kashefi F, Khajehei M, Alavinia M, Golmakani E, Asili J. Effect of ginger (Zingiber officinale) on heavy menstrual bleeding: a placebo-controlled, randomized clinical trial. Phytother Res. 2015 Jan;29(1):114-9. https://pubmed.ncbi.nlm.nih.gov/25298352/
78. Ghalandari S, Kariman N, Sheikhan Z, Mojab F, Mirzaei M, Shahrahmani H. Effect of Hydroalcoholic Extract of Capsella bursa pastoris on Early Postpartum Hemorrhage: A Clinical Trial Study. J Altern Complement Med. 2017 Oct;23(10):794-799. https://pubmed.ncbi.nlm.nih.gov/28590768/
79. Naafe M, Kariman N, Keshavarz Z, Khademi N, Mojab F, Mohammadbeigi A. Effect of Hydroalcoholic Extracts of Capsella Bursa-Pastoris on Heavy Menstrual Bleeding: A Randomized Clinical Trial. J Altern Complement Med. 2018 Jul;24(7):694-700. https://pubmed.ncbi.nlm.nih.gov/29641247/
80. Choi WJ, Kim SK, Park HK, Sohn UD, Kim W. Anti-Inflammatory and Anti-Superbacterial Properties of Sulforaphane from Shepherd's Purse. Korean J Physiol Pharmacol. 2014 Feb;18(1):33-9. https://www.ncbi.nlm.nih.gov/pmc/articles/PMC3951821/#
81. Ghorbani A, Esmaeilizadeh M. Pharmacological properties of *Salvia officinalis* and its components. J Tradit Complement Med. 2017 Jan 13;7(4):433-440. https://www.ncbi.nlm.nih.gov/pmc/articles/PMC5634728/
82. Lee KB, Cho E, Kang YS. Changes in 5-hydroxytryptamine and cortisol plasma levels in menopausal women after inhalation of clary sage oil. Phytother Res. 2014 Nov;28(11):1599-605. https://www.ncbi.nlm.nih.gov/pubmed/24802524
83. Bommer S, Klein P, Suter A. First time proof of sage's tolerability and efficacy in menopausal women with hot flushes. Adv Ther. 2011 Jun;28(6):490-500. https://www.ncbi.nlm.nih.gov/pubmed/21630133
84. Avelino-Flores Mdel C, Cruz-López Mdel C, Jiménez-Montejo FE, Reyes-Leyva J. Cytotoxic activity of the methanolic extract of Turnera

diffusa Willd on breast cancer cells. J Med Food. 2015 Mar;18(3):299-305. https://pubmed.ncbi.nlm.nih.gov/25299247/
85. Meddah B, Ducroc R, El Abbes Faouzi M, Eto B, Mahraoui L, Benhaddou-Andaloussi A, Martineau LC, Cherrah Y, Haddad PS. Nigella sativa inhibits intestinal glucose absorption and improves glucose tolerance in rats. J Ethnopharmacol. 2009 Jan 30;121(3):419-24. https://pubmed.ncbi.nlm.nih.gov/19061948/
86. Abo El-Magd NF, El-Mesery M, El-Karef A, El-Shishtawy MM. Amelioration effect of black seed oil against high-fat diet-induced obesity in rats through Nrf2/HO-1 pathway. J Food Biochem. 2021 Apr;45(4):e13693. https://pubmed.ncbi.nlm.nih.gov/33719073/
87. Najmi A, Nasiruddin M, Khan RA, Haque SF. Effect of Nigella sativa oil on various clinical and biochemical parameters of insulin resistance syndrome. Int J Diabetes Dev Ctries. 2008 Jan;28(1):11-4. https://www.ncbi.nlm.nih.gov/pmc/articles/PMC2772004/
88. Bin Sayeed MS, Shams T, Fahim Hossain S, Rahman MR, Mostofa A, Fahim Kadir M, Mahmood S, Asaduzzaman M. Nigella sativa L. seeds modulate mood, anxiety and cognition in healthy adolescent males. J Ethnopharmacol. 2014 Feb 27;152(1):156-62. https://pubmed.ncbi.nlm.nih.gov/24412554/
89. Farhangi MA, Dehghan P, Tajmiri S, Abbasi MM. The effects of Nigella sativa on thyroid function, serum Vascular Endothelial Growth Factor (VEGF) - 1, Nesfatin-1 and anthropometric features in patients with Hashimoto's thyroiditis: a randomized controlled trial. BMC Complement Altern Med. 2016 Nov 16;16(1):471. https://pubmed.ncbi.nlm.nih.gov/27852303/
90. Parhizkar S, Latiff LA, Parsa A. Effect of Nigella sativa on reproductive system in experimental menopause rat model. Avicenna J Phytomed. 2016 Jan-Feb;6(1):95-103. https://www.ncbi.nlm.nih.gov/pmc/articles/PMC4884222/
91. Heydarpour F, Hemati N, Hadi A, Moradi S, Mohammadi E, Farzaei MH. Effects of cinnamon on controlling metabolic parameters of polycystic ovary syndrome: A systematic review and meta-analysis. J

Ethnopharmacol. 2020 May 23;254:112741. https://pubmed.ncbi.nlm.nih.gov/32151755/#

92. Zarezadeh M, Musazadeh V, Foroumandi E, Keramati M, Ostadrahimi A, Mekary RA. The effect of cinnamon supplementation on glycemic control in patients with type 2 diabetes or with polycystic ovary syndrome: an umbrella meta-analysis on interventional meta-analyses. Diabetol Metab Syndr. 2023 Jun 15;15(1):127. https://pubmed.ncbi.nlm.nih.gov/37316893/

93. Jaafarpour M, Hatefi M, Najafi F, Khajavikhan J, Khani A. The effect of cinnamon on menstrual bleeding and systemic symptoms with primary dysmenorrhea. Iran Red Crescent Med J. 2015 Apr 22;17(4):e27032. https://pubmed.ncbi.nlm.nih.gov/26023350/

94. Cai, B., Zhang, Y., Wang, Z., Xu, D., Jia, Y., Guan, Y., Liao, A., Liu, G., Chun, C., & Li, J. (2020). Therapeutic potential of diosgenin and its major derivatives against neurological diseases: Recent advances. *Oxidative Medicine and Cellular Longevity, 2020*, 1–16. https://www.hindawi.com/journals/omcl/2020/3153082/

95. Park MK, Kwon HY, Ahn WS, Bae S, Rhyu MR, Lee Y. Estrogen activities and the cellular effects of natural progesterone from wild yam extract in mcf-7 human breast cancer cells. Am J Chin Med. 2009;37(1):159-67. https://pubmed.ncbi.nlm.nih.gov/19222119/

96. Final report of the amended safety assessment of Dioscorea Villosa (Wild Yam) root extract. Int J Toxicol. 2004;23 Suppl 2:49-54. https://pubmed.ncbi.nlm.nih.gov/15513824/

97. Bhandari MR, Kawabata J. Bitterness and toxicity in wild yam (Dioscorea spp.) tubers of Nepal. Plant Foods Hum Nutr. 2005 Sep;60(3):129-35. https://pubmed.ncbi.nlm.nih.gov/16187016/

98. Oh SM, Chung KH. Antiestrogenic activities of Ginkgo biloba extracts. J Steroid Biochem Mol Biol. 2006 Aug;100(4-5):167-76. https://pubmed.ncbi.nlm.nih.gov/16842996/

99. Fang J, Wang Z, Wang P, Wang M. Extraction, structure and bioactivities of the polysaccharides from Ginkgo biloba: A review. Int J Biol Macromol. 2020 Nov 1;162:1897-1905. https://pubmed.ncbi.nlm.ni

h.gov/32827622/
100. Tamborini A, Taurelle R. Intérêt de l'extrait standardisé de Ginkgo biloba (EGb 761) dans la prise en charge des symptômes congestifs du syndrome prémenstruel [Value of standardized Ginkgo biloba extract (EGb 761) in the management of congestive symptoms of premenstrual syndrome]. Rev Fr Gynecol Obstet. 1993 Jul-Sep;88(7-9):447-57. French. https://pubmed.ncbi.nlm.nih.gov/8235261/
101. Ozgoli G, Selselei EA, Mojab F, Majd HA. A randomized, placebo-controlled trial of Ginkgo biloba L. in treatment of premenstrual syndrome. J Altern Complement Med. 2009 Aug;15(8):845-51. https://pubmed.ncbi.nlm.nih.gov/19678774/
102. Mix JA, Crews WD Jr. A double-blind, placebo-controlled, randomized trial of Ginkgo biloba extract EGb 761 in a sample of cognitively intact older adults: neuropsychological findings. Hum Psychopharmacol. 2002 Aug;17(6):267-77. https://pubmed.ncbi.nlm.nih.gov/12404671/
103. Savaskan E, Mueller H, Hoerr R, von Gunten A, Gauthier S. Treatment effects of Ginkgo biloba extract EGb 761® on the spectrum of behavioral and psychological symptoms of dementia: meta-analysis of randomized controlled trials. Int Psychogeriatr. 2018 Mar;30(3):285-293. https://pubmed.ncbi.nlm.nih.gov/28931444/
104. Bhusal KK, Magar SK, Thapa R, Lamsal A, Bhandari S, Maharjan R, Shrestha S, Shrestha J. Nutritional and pharmacological importance of stinging nettle (*Urtica dioica* L.): A review. Heliyon. 2022 Jun 22;8(6):e09717. https://www.ncbi.nlm.nih.gov/pmc/articles/PMC9253158/
105. Kargozar R, Salari R, Jarahi L, Yousefi M, Pourhoseini SA, Sahebkar-Khorasani M, Azizi H. Urtica dioica in comparison with placebo and acupuncture: A new possibility for menopausal hot flashes: A randomized clinical trial. Complement Ther Med. 2019 Jun;44:166-173. https://pubmed.ncbi.nlm.nih.gov/31126551/
106. Karimi FZ, Nazari N, Rakhshandeh H, Mazloum SR. The effect of nettle vaginal cream on subjective symptoms of vaginal atrophy in

postmenopausal women. Eur J Obstet Gynecol Reprod Biol. 2023 Jun;285:41-45. https://pubmed.ncbi.nlm.nih.gov/37044017/
107. Liu L, Li H, Tan G, Ma Z. Traditional Chinese herbal medicine in treating amenorrhea caused by antipsychotic drugs: Meta-analysis and systematic review. J Ethnopharmacol. 2022 May 10;289:115044. https://pubmed.ncbi.nlm.nih.gov/35101572/
108. Fung FY, Wong WH, Ang SK, Koh HL, Kun MC, Lee LH, Li X, Ng HJ, Tan CW, Zhao Y, Linn YC. A randomized, double-blind, placebo-controlled study on the anti-haemostatic effects of Curcuma longa, Angelica sinensis and Panax ginseng. Phytomedicine. 2017 Aug 15;32:88-96. https://pubmed.ncbi.nlm.nih.gov/28732813/
109. Kupfersztain C, Rotem C, Fagot R, Kaplan B. The immediate effect of natural plant extract, Angelica sinensis and Matricaria chamomilla (Climex) for the treatment of hot flushes during menopause. A preliminary report. Clin Exp Obstet Gynecol. 2003;30(4):203-6. https://pubmed.ncbi.nlm.nih.gov/14664413/
110. Zhu H, You J, Wen Y, Jia L, Gao F, Ganesan K, Chen J. Tumorigenic risk of Angelica sinensis on ER-positive breast cancer growth through ER-induced stemness in vitro and in vivo. J Ethnopharmacol. 2021 Nov 15;280:114415. https://pubmed.ncbi.nlm.nih.gov/34271113/
111. Chiu SC, Chiu TL, Huang SY, Chang SF, Chen SP, Pang CY, Hsieh TF. Potential therapeutic effects of N-butylidenephthalide from Radix Angelica Sinensis (Danggui) in human bladder cancer cells. BMC Complement Altern Med. 2017 Dec 6;17(1):523. https://pubmed.ncbi.nlm.nih.gov/29207978/
112. Wang C, Lv X, Liu W, Liu S, Sun Z. Uncovering the pharmacological mechanism of motherwort (Leonurus japonicus Houtt.) for treating menstrual disorders: A systems pharmacology approach. Comput Biol Chem. 2020 Dec;89:107384. https://pubmed.ncbi.nlm.nih.gov/33017723/
113. Liu W, Ma S, Pan W, Tan W. Combination of motherwort injection and oxytocin for the prevention of postpartum hemorrhage after cesarean section. J Matern Fetal Neonatal Med. 2016;29(15):2490-3. https://p

ubmed.ncbi.nlm.nih.gov/26414626/
114. Shikov AN, Pozharitskaya ON, Makarov VG, Demchenko DV, Shikh EV. Effect of Leonurus cardiaca oil extract in patients with arterial hypertension accompanied by anxiety and sleep disorders. Phytother Res. 2011 Apr;25(4):540-3. https://pubmed.ncbi.nlm.nih.gov/20839214/
115. Koshovyi O, Raal A, Kireyev I, Tryshchuk N, Ilina T, Romanenko Y, Kovalenko SM, Bunyatyan N. Phytochemical and Psychotropic Research of Motherwort (*Leonurus cardiaca* L.) Modified Dry Extracts. Plants (Basel). 2021 Jan 25;10(2):230. https://pubmed.ncbi.nlm.nih.gov/33503956/
116. Bernatoniene J, Kopustinskiene DM, Jakstas V, Majiene D, Baniene R, Kuršvietiene L, Masteikova R, Savickas A, Toleikis A, Trumbeckaite S. The effect of Leonurus cardiaca herb extract and some of its flavonoids on mitochondrial oxidative phosphorylation in the heart. Planta Med. 2014 May;80(7):525-32. https://pubmed.ncbi.nlm.nih.gov/24841965/
117. Fierascu RC, Fierascu I, Ortan A, Fierascu IC, Anuta V, Velescu BS, Pituru SM, Dinu-Pirvu CE. *Leonurus cardiaca* L. as a Source of Bioactive Compounds: An Update of the European Medicines Agency Assessment Report (2010). Biomed Res Int. 2019 Apr 17;2019:4303215. https://www.ncbi.nlm.nih.gov/pmc/articles/PMC6500680/
118. Fierascu RC, Fierascu I, Ortan A, Fierascu IC, Anuta V, Velescu BS, Pituru SM, Dinu-Pirvu CE. *Leonurus cardiaca* L. as a Source of Bioactive Compounds: An Update of the European Medicines Agency Assessment Report (2010). Biomed Res Int. 2019 Apr 17;2019:4303215. https://pubmed.ncbi.nlm.nih.gov/22049281/
119. Janda K, Wojtkowska K, Jakubczyk K, Antoniewicz J, Skonieczna-Żydecka K. *Passiflora incarnata* in Neuropsychiatric Disorders-A Systematic Review. Nutrients. 2020 Dec 19;12(12):3894. https://www.ncbi.nlm.nih.gov/pmc/articles/PMC7766837/
120. Nojoumi M, Ghaeli P, Salimi S, Sharifi A, Raisi F. Effects of Passion

Flower Extract, as an Add-On Treatment to Sertraline, on Reaction Time in Patients with Generalized Anxiety Disorder: A Double-Blind Placebo-Controlled Study. Iran J Psychiatry. 2016 Jul;11(3):191-197. https://www.ncbi.nlm.nih.gov/pmc/articles/PMC5139955/

121. Guerrero FA, Medina GM. Effect of a medicinal plant (*Passiflora incarnata* L) on sleep. Sleep Sci. 2017 Jul-Sep;10(3):96-100. https://www.ncbi.nlm.nih.gov/pmc/articles/PMC5699852/

122. Wang T, Xue B, Shao H, Wang SY, Bai L, Yin CH, Zhao HY, Qi YC, Cui LL, He X, Ma YM. Effect of Dandelion Extracts on the Proliferation of Ovarian Granulosa Cells and Expression of Hormone Receptors. Chin Med J (Engl). 2018 Jul 20;131(14):1694-1701. https://www.ncbi.nlm.nih.gov/pmc/articles/PMC6048925/

123. Oh SM, Kim HR, Park YJ, Lee YH, Chung KH. Ethanolic extract of dandelion (Taraxacum mongolicum) induces estrogenic activity in MCF-7 cells and immature rats. Chin J Nat Med. 2015 Nov;13(11):808-814. https://pubmed.ncbi.nlm.nih.gov/26614455/

124. Clare BA, Conroy RS, Spelman K. The diuretic effect in human subjects of an extract of Taraxacum officinale folium over a single day. J Altern Complement Med. 2009 Aug;15(8):929-34. https://pubmed.ncbi.nlm.nih.gov/19678785

125. Fan M, Zhang X, Song H, Zhang Y. Dandelion (*Taraxacum* Genus): A Review of Chemical Constituents and Pharmacological Effects. Molecules. 2023 Jun 27;28(13):5022. https://www.ncbi.nlm.nih.gov/pmc/articles/PMC10343869/

126. Pfingstgraf IO, Taulescu M, Pop RM, Orăsan R, Vlase L, Uifalean A, Todea D, Alexescu T, Toma C, Pârvu AE. Protective Effects of *Taraxacum officinale* L. (Dandelion) Root Extract in Experimental Acute on Chronic Liver Failure. Antioxidants (Basel). 2021 Mar 24;10(4):504. https://www.ncbi.nlm.nih.gov/pmc/articles/PMC8063808/

127. *British Herbal Pharmacopoeia 1996*. (1996). . British Herbal Medicine Association. https://bhma.info/product/british-herbal-pharmacopoeia-1996/

128. Estrada-Reyes R, Carro-Juárez M, Martínez-Mota L. Pro-sexual effects

of Turnera diffusa Wild (Turneraceae) in male rats involves the nitric oxide pathway. J Ethnopharmacol. 2013 Mar 7;146(1):164-72. https://pubmed.ncbi.nlm.nih.gov/23298455/

129. Taha MM, Salga MS, Ali HM, Abdulla MA, Abdelwahab SI, Hadi AH. Gastroprotective activities of Turnera diffusa Willd. ex Schult. revisited: Role of arbutin. J Ethnopharmacol. 2012 May 7;141(1):273-81. https://pubmed.ncbi.nlm.nih.gov/22374081/

130. Zhao J, Dasmahapatra AK, Khan SI, Khan IA. Anti-aromatase activity of the constituents from damiana (Turnera diffusa). J Ethnopharmacol. 2008 Dec 8;120(3):387-93. https://pubmed.ncbi.nlm.nih.gov/18948180/

131. Taha MM, Salga MS, Ali HM, Abdulla MA, Abdelwahab SI, Hadi AH. Gastroprotective activities of Turnera diffusa Willd. ex Schult. revisited: Role of arbutin. J Ethnopharmacol. 2012 May 7;141(1):273-81. http://www.ncbi.nlm.nih.gov/pubmed/22374081

132. Avelino-Flores Mdel C, Cruz-López Mdel C, Jiménez-Montejo FE, Reyes-Leyva J. Cytotoxic activity of the methanolic extract of Turnera diffusa Willd on breast cancer cells. J Med Food. 2015 Mar;18(3):299-305. https://www.ncbi.nlm.nih.gov/pmc/articles/PMC4350145/

Six

Chapter 6

Special Period Concerns

Menstrual cycles are often anything but normal for an alarming number of women. In fact, almost all women I talk to have some major physical or mental symptoms around their periods, but it doesn't have to be that way.

In this chapter, I review some common period issues that can be at least partially but sometimes fully addressed using natural diet and supplement approaches and herbal therapies. Included in this chapter is an evaluation of natural versus synthetic hormone replacement. Then, I explain my own journey to healing from mid-cycle ovarian pain, heavy periods, painful periods, and irregular periods. I also explore the root causes of endometriosis and polycystic ovarian syndrome that plague so many women and how to naturally reduce the symptoms of these conditions.

Still, you should always be evaluated by your healthcare provider if you have heavy bleeding, any type of women's pain, or changes in your cycle that are unexplained by typical things like stress or diet fluctuations. And please do get your yearly checkups. But I highly encourage you to have a conversation about natural therapies with your provider. If they seem reluctant to talk about these areas, you might want to get a second opinion.

Don't worry, I will get into premenstrual syndrome, perimenopausal, menopausal symptoms, and menstrual migraines in Chapter 7.

Bioidentical Progesterone for Perimenopause, Heavy Periods, and PCOS

Bioidentical progesterone is different from synthetic progesterone found in prescription hormones. Yet major health websites deem bioidentical progesterone as having identical risks despite clear research evidence to the contrary[1-9]. Natural progesterone is often derived from wild yams, and you see, no money is to be made from wild yams. Thus, the websites that have a lot of money to gain from people filling yet another prescription, which are almost all major health websites. These cites downplay any potential benefit of natural over synthetic. Shockingly, I found 8 research studies and 1 review study of 6 clinical trials stating the clear benefits and safety of using **bioidentical** progesterone for women and indeed a clear reduction in cancer risk over synthetic hormones.[1-9] I don't know if and when these major websites will ever be held accountable for spreading false information but I hope someday they are.

Moving on to what people use bioidentical progesterone from wild yams for. This type of progesterone is identical to the progesterone that our bodies make and for this reason, it doesn't carry the same risks of synthetic hormones. As you may recall, low progesterone levels in the body forces the body to become estrogen dominant and causes too much bleeding or abnormal bleeding. Many women are estrogen dominant, including those with fertility issues like PCOS, perimenopausal women, and women with imbalanced diets and lots of stress. This captures a large percentage of women who are low in this protective hormone. While I'm not suggesting that women's first step should be to grab some bioidentical progesterone to cover this up, there is a time and a place for using this natural therapy and PCOS and perimenopause may be that place. Bioidentical progesterone helps improve fertility in women with PCOS and offers clear symptom relief for women in perimenopause including a reduction in heavy bleeding. On a personal note, natural progesterone cream, along with wild yam cream, has made a dramatic difference for me in my perimenopausal years for reducing abnormal bleeding. It is the difference between me getting a hysterectomy and naturally easing into menopause feeling stronger and healthier with natural progesterone and wild yam among my other herbal remedies. I've seen women go the hysterectomy route and live to regret this decision for the rest of their lives due to the complications of the surgery.

It is always smart to see your healthcare provider if you have excess bleeding during perimenopause, but if your provider doesn't at this point offer you bioidentical progesterone before a hysterectomy for simple low progesterone levels that causes heavy bleeding you should seek out a second opinion. While you can get your hormones checked during perimenopause, please know that hormones swing wildly with no rhyme or reason so it may not always be that helpful in some women to do so. You can get bioidentical progesterone as a prescription or also as a topical cream which is sold over-the-counter. I suggest checking with your provider to help navigate timing and dosages. I personally love and use Emerita Pro-Gest which is known as "the original balancing cream." This is a topical progesterone that requires only about a dime-sized drop of the cream applied to your skin. And it's available in health food stores and on the internet. Most women find that it helps reduce abnormal bleeding in as little as 3 days but I found that it reduces my abnormal bleeding within 1 day.

What About Bioidentical Estrogen?

Contrary to what the internet might try to tell you, bioidentical estrogen also is safer than synthetic estrogen because it is in the more neutral estriol form we reviewed in Chapter 2. It doesn't increase the risk of blood clots like synthetic estradiol and bioidentical estrogen all the while improves cardiovascular health markers along with improved mood and sexual function.[10-12] But before using bioidentical estrogen, I highly suggest that you get your hormones tested because estrogen coming from any form needs to be dosed carefully and can cause more bleeding if you are already doing well making your own estrogen.

Mid-Cycle Ovarian Pain

Mid-cycle ovarian pain, aka Mittelschmerz, according to authoritative websites and my doctor at the time of my issue, has no known causes. Most medical websites say to just take birth control. Huh? No known causes but just throw birth control at it? Fun! A pill with tons of side effects and that robs the body of lots of nutrients? Sounds like the sort of terrible advice for almost everything out there if you have a women's problem. Sadly, this advice doesn't get to the root problem and likely only makes things worse in the long run!

After the birth of my daughter, not only were my periods awful, I ended up getting pain in my left ovary from ovulation through the end of my period for months on end. This meant I was in pain half of my life. Like I mentioned earlier, I went to the doctor, and they told me I had Mittelschmerz after doing an ultrasound. Mittelschmerz has no known causes, or so they say, and it's just a name to describe mid-cycle pain. They told me to take ibuprofen since I can't take the pill. This was tired and unhelpful advice. And potentially very harmful advice if you take ibuprofen for half of the month year in and year out. So, this fueled my frustration and that very day, I walked out of the doctor's office and into the herbal store looking for a better way and I found it.

By luck, I found the perfect solution right away. I had a strong basis for knowledge of supplements in general, and I found a supplement containing DIM (broccoli compound), calcium D-glucarate (also a broccoli compound), rosemary, milk thistle, turmeric, and another form of broccoli sprout extract. After taking this natural supplement for just one month, my pain went away, and it did another amazing thing: it gave me the root cause of what is going on in reverse and I'll explain that soon. Let me repeat that, my pain was gone, not just reduced, by adding in a safe and natural supplement. I was blown away! It also reduced my period pain. What an amazing find! And the pain stayed away as long as I stayed on this concoction and my period pain significantly reduced too. Later, I learned that eating raw broccoli every day accomplished the same thing, along with eating other broccoli family foods. I'm still sad that the supplement called Estrosense I found at the time is harder to find at this point. But you can find it directly from the website called Natural Factors and I recommend that you do so. It also is available on Instacart.

Back to the root cause of mid-cycle ovarian pain, at least for me. Calcium D-glucarate is a natural compound found in the broccoli family of vegetables and this is a hormone-detoxifying compound just like broccoli sprout extract is.[13-14] My mid-cycle pain was due to a lack of proper detoxification of hormones. AHA! The best part is that this supplement combination is very safe because it comes from broccoli (and also smells like broccoli). While this exact supplement isn't easy to find, you can easily find a calcium-D glucarate and broccoli supplement, such as those called DIM complex supplements available on Fullscript like Pure Encapsulations DIM detox.

By matter of logic, it appears to me that Mittelschmerz is caused by improper estrogen metabolism by the liver and gut. Simply adding in estrogen-detoxing broccoli fixed the issue. It makes me wonder how many other women's issues have this simple fix that are fully not discussed or researched?

If you have ovarian pain which they can't find a cause for, this is certainly a safe thing to try. Other things you could try that also help with hormone balance are herbs like dandelion root and vitex, raspberry leaf, turmeric, ginger, and milk thistle. These boost antioxidants in the body while also helping the liver to break down harmful compounds including toxic forms of estrogen as reviewed in Chapter 2.

Heavy Periods

> *"I bleed twelve weeks a year, so I know a thing or two about bloodstains."*
> — **Amanda Lovelace, The Witch Doesn't Burn in This One**

Having a horribly heavy period isn't necessarily something you will have forever if you strengthen your uterus with herbs and nutrients. A stronger uterus means it is less likely to bleed heavily due to a weak lining. While you may not have the delicate periods that some women have, you can stop the raging river naturally in many cases, so to speak. And I learned to do so by scouring the Library of Medicine with a fine-toothed comb and with the help of my naturopath.

It can't be said enough that you should seek help from your healthcare provider if you struggle with heavy periods to rule out anything serious before embarking on tips I suggest below and review these with your provider before trying them.

As discussed in Chapter 3, if you are low in iron, this weakens the lining of the uterus, making it so your periods are heavy. **What kind of bullshit is**

Chapter 6

that? But, this means there is also a solution; in my experience, you can't fall off of supplementing iron and expect your periods to stay lighter. You have to commit to taking it regularly.

Along with iron as reviewed on page 59, you should seriously consider eating beef liver or supplementing beef liver regularly and/or take vitamin A as well. Ladies, if you have had heavy periods, your uterus has been depleted for a long time! A personal note about beef liver: I struggle to cook it at home because not everyone in the house is on board with eating it, however I do sneak it in when I can. But to get it on a consistent basis, I absolutely need to supplement beef liver capsules. If I don't, I notice that my menstrual cycle is noticeably heavier. It's one supplement that I can't move away from. You may also need to eat your beef liver daily if you suffer from heavy periods!

Some other nutrients for a heavy period that you can take to help are vitamin E, vitamin C, and vitamin K2 are important too as reviewed in Chapter 3. Getting on a supplement that supports progesterone is also a good idea such as herbs like Vitex and dandelion root. Progesterone strengthens the uterus. For many years, I've been taking an herbal combination with these compounds in them called Vitanica Women's Phase I which you can find at a local herbal store, health store, or at their website directly. It can prove to be difficult to find sometimes because it is in high demand and the manufacturer can't keep up. Adding Shepherd's purse as described on page 108 will slow a heavy flow. Using other herbs that help reduce bleeding amount include ginger, turmeric, and red raspberry leaf can be life-changing for many women with heavy periods. Just don't expect them to work overnight; you need to incorporate healthy herbs like these 3 regularly for them to work.

As I inch closer to menopause, adding in daily vitex supplement, DHEA, and tribulus are helpful too for reducing my period burden. I also use some topical wild yam and some natural progesterone called Pro-gest by Emerita as mentioned previously. This can help younger women too who struggle with estrogen dominance. These remedies are nothing short of a miracle for many women, so I encourage you to dabble in them once you have been evaluated by your healthcare provider.

Painful Periods

> "Cramps aren't that bad? Neither is a punch in the crotch."
> **-Unkown**

Many of the tips listed to help with mid-cycle pain and heavy periods also apply to reducing the chances of painful periods. However, there is more research devoted to reducing period pain, so there are many other tools you can use to help ease your menstrual pain naturally. I will list these in order of how I find them to be effective. But they are all helpful in their own way and safe if used correctly according to the package directions, so you could try multiples at a time, which I do recommend. But please consult with your healthcare provider if you have period pain to rule out anything that may need medical attention.

Remember that these supplements can't replace a healthy eating plan, so try to incorporate as many tips from the recipes and meal planning sections of this book as possible too.

Did you know....CBD Suppositories Reduce Menstrual Pain

I hesitated to include this tip, but timing is everything. For one of the most effective period pain relievers, I simply add cannabis tincture onto the top of my tampons, making it a medical suppository. It works almost instantly to reduce the pain of periods. While I was getting this book ready to publish, a study proved my theory that full-spectrum CBD oil suppositories do indeed reduce pain, improve mood, and reduce the need for pain medications[15]. You see, sometimes instincts are right and with herbs, I trusted my instincts. I want to thank my good friend Cheryl for showing me this new piece of research!

Broccoli supplements are my first love when it comes to reducing horrible menstrual pain. They took me from the equivalent of stabbing sharp pains all the time to much more mild and manageable cramps. If you focus on eating raw broccoli every day, you may not need to supplement broccoli. Bear in mind that the research hasn't yet vetted this out, but it's been my consistent experience that broccoli simply works to reduce period pain and ovarian pain because it improves estrogen ratios in the body as discussed on page 37.

Vitex helps to naturally increase progesterone and support normal ovulation, which ultimately can reduce your period pain. This may take a few months to work, but in my case, it worked much more quickly to help especially when I combine it with motherwort.

Vitamin A, boron, and iron are indispensable for building a healthy uterus. They are most critical to take if you have heavy periods, which can leave you severely low in both vitamin A and iron. Ironically, taking both can strengthen your uterus which ultimately results in less period pain too in my experience and according to research. Boron helps reduce period pain too.

Motherwort is a fascinating herb that is heart-protective as well as a uterine tonic. As such, it can help ease your period pain too. The verdict is still out about whether or not it reduces period bleeding volume, but I certainly find that for me it reduces large blood clots and abdominal pain. The combination of vitex and motherwort works great for me for reducing period pain as I get closer to menopause.

Pine bark is effective for all kinds of pain and that includes period pain.

Vitanica Women's Phase I has been an indispensable supplement for me and is so popular, it sells out. It's a blend of herbs and vitamins that reduces menstrual pain.

CBD:THC in a 1:1 ratio: Cannabis is a great natural pain reliever. For period pain, I suggest getting an edible tincture or flower that is 50% CBD because of its ability to reduce pain. It's also great for promoting healthy sleep. When using this ratio, you also will be less likely to feel "high." But do what works best for you because we all respond a bit differently to cannabinoids.

Vitamin E helps period pain by dampening inflammation. A dose of 150-400 IU per day is enough to make a difference as reviewed on page 71, but just be sure to be patient and give it at least 2 months to work. If you take Vitanica Women's Phase I you won't need any extra vitamin E.

Thiamine safely helps with inflammation and reduces pain signals, so it's a no-brainer to try for pain, but also be patient-it takes 2 months to work. Taking 100 mg per day is a safe and effective dose. You can also combine with other B-vitamins by using a natural B complex to ensure you are getting a balance of B vitamins.

Vitamin C helps detoxify hormones and also decreases inflammation-related pain while also decreasing allergy symptoms as reviewed on page 64. Supplemental vitamin C will always be part of my life for all of these reasons!

Calcium, Magnesium, and Zinc these calming minerals help to reduce symptoms of period pain. Make sure to try to get the calcium and zinc from your diet so that you only really need to supplement magnesium. But if you are vegetarian or vegan or avoid red meat and seafood, getting enough zinc is nearly impossible because it's not very bioavailable from plants. In this case, supplementing zinc may help your period pain. If you avoid dairy, it's also very difficult to get calcium, so you still may need a calcium supplement to help reduce menstrual cramps.

Chapter 6

Irregular Periods

As I discussed at the beginning of the book, a regular period is a bit of an oxymoron and is more a unicorn than a real thing. After all, a "normal" period can be from 24-38 days apart and 2-8 days long. But a period isn't "normal" or if you lose more or less blood than "usual". Seems a bit suspect if you ask me.

Coming from a person who got a hot and heavy period like clockwork every 24-28 days for most of my life, this section took a little more of a deep dive into the research. However, you should know that heavy periods, or too light for that matter, are technically irregular too so I guess I join the ranks as irregular like everyone else. But, there are some things you can do if you have majorly irregular periods once you figure out the cause of your irregular cycles.

You should know that irregular periods can have many different causes. Common causes of irregular periods are PCOS, breastfeeding, hormonal birth control, IUDs, perimenopause, thyroid disorders, eating disorders, endometriosis, Celiac disease, diabetes, and other rare conditions. It's important to figure out the underlying causes of irregular periods with your healthcare provider.

Beyond that, there are a lot of things you can do to be proactive with herbal and food remedies as well as careful exercise as reviewed throughout this book.

As a general rule, exercise, but don't overdo it, if you want to help fix your irregular periods. Many women don't know that too much exercise can cause your periods to be irregular and can rob you of sex drive. This is more common than people realize because of the push for exercise at all costs in our society. For more information, learn about your Inner Seasons on page 24.

Of course, if you are breastfeeding or pregnant it is normal to lose your period and this is a time you can relish in skipping periods. Yay! Well, unless you are like me and got your period right away despite breastfeeding my babies. My uterus really likes to produce periods!

In the next sections, you will learn how to manage irregular periods that are caused by low or high thyroid levels, eating disorders, and more. See Page 163 for tips about PCOS and Page 154 for tips about endometriosis-related irregular periods.

Ways to Cope With Eating Disorders

It goes without saying that if you have an eating disorder, you should seek out a counselor and doctor who specializes in this topic and seek hospitalization if you are at a severe stage of your eating disorder.

That said, I worked with people who had eating disorders for more than 15 years when I worked in a hospital and I can tell you quite a few things that I learned along the way from research and from my patients.

Using guided meditation or a reputable clinical hypnotherapist are two of my top recommendations for anyone going through the difficulties of eating disorders. A review in Psychology Today concluded that meditation indeed helps with eating disorder recovery.[16] Clinical hypnotherapy is a great tool that helps you to more effectively meditate on your own and bring calm to mealtimes. If this isn't accessible or doesn't feel right for you, it is also possible to find guided meditation/self hypnosis on YouTube and I recommend checking out Michael Seeley's channel where he helps guide you through this safely and easily.

Often in clinical practice, I would do guided meditation with patients by

Chapter 6

having them visualize in their mind's eye a simple image of something, perhaps a pet or nature, and have them describe how picturing this image in their mind could bring a sense of calm in the brain. I would have them do this every time they would eat and it was effective in helping them eat and be more accepting of food.

Working from the framework of healing and supporting vitality with nutrients is often a more appealing tool for people struggling with eating disorders as opposed to cramming in calories and locking the bathroom door as is done in many hospitalized settings for eating disorders. And while intuitive eating is popular in eating disorder recovery circles which can be helpful, it doesn't always get to the root of eating issues or period issues for that matter.

I'm an example of how healing the gut may do as much, if not more, than forcing calories in for normalizing a menstrual cycle and normalizing weight. As you may recall, my periods were irregular in that they were too heavy and too painful. During my teens and twenties, I was also pretty underweight and struggled to gain weight. Most people couldn't believe how much food I could eat without gaining weight! I would often get accused of having an eating disorder even though I did not; my eating disorder was eating a lot and not absorbing it as it turns out! I would eat more than everyone around me. But, this actually was a problem. I should have known that my gut wasn't absorbing things well, but back in the day, science knew very little about food intolerances and food sensitivities. While I didn't have an eating disorder in the classical sense, I had a lot of anxiety and gut troubles back before I knew what was causing what in my body. Desperate to get pregnant, I would eat copious amounts of just about anything so that I could gain enough weight to be pregnant. I finally did gain enough weight to get pregnant, but I still had the underlying gut and anxiety troubles. At age 38 I finally turned to functional medicine and learned that most of my troubles with anxiety and my too low of body weight stemmed from gluten sensitivity. A lot of my anxiety stemmed from gluten too, because it put my immune system on high alert all the time.

But, I didn't truly get a full handle on my anxiety until I went to a good clinical hypnotherapist and took some amino acid supplements that helped balance my mood. Hypnotherapy is ridiculously misunderstood because of dumb sideshows at fairs. In my opinion it is the most effective tool that helps you learn to meditate well on your own.

And yes, I know what you are thinking: amino acids come from protein, so just eat more protein. In a perfect world yes. I do truly eat a lot of protein but this doesn't mean that my body makes enough dopamine from these foods: I needed tyrosine to make dopamine and my body needed more serotonin from tryptophan. I learned about tyrosine with the help of a good friend and colleague of mine and I've been taking it along with tryptophan for years to help regulate my mood. If you haven't tried these two things, I highly recommend that you do, and the supplement Neurolink has a good balance of the two nutrients: tyrosine to tryptophan in a 10:1 ratio. I suggest starting at half the dose that the bottle recommends. While this supplement doesn't help everyone, there is a good chance it will help you if you are low in amino acids. And if you have an eating disorder, the odds are, you are low in these amino acids and just about every other nutrient.

This is why I also recommend ruling out food intolerances and sensitivities for eating disorders because they can mask the underlying reasons you are not able to eat well and gain weight as well as have normal periods. I also recommend healing the gut with probiotics. After all, gut disturbances from food intolerances can even make you afraid to eat from the pain it causes.

Then, in order to restore and heal your gut, you will want to replace the missing nutrients with a good broad-spectrum natural multivitamin with mineral supplement such as Pure Encapsulations brand. I also suggest taking extra thiamine to restore your gut lining along with bovine colostrum for gut healing and adding boron supplements to help normalize hormones. If you are willing, you should also incorporate organ meats into your diet on a regular basis because they are nature's best multivitamin. Have your doctor check your ferritin levels because, odds are, you are low in iron if you have an eating disorder. Last but not least, motherwort herb can help restore normal menstrual cycles in some women as reviewed on page 116.

You might also want to try to eat a healing diet as described in Chapter 8.

Natural Thyroid Remedies for Irregular Periods

A lot of people don't realize that if they have abnormal thyroid levels it can cause abnormal periods. The face behind the mask of all of these thyroid and period issues is often food sensitivities and food allergies along with inadequate vitamins, antioxidants, protein, fats, and minerals.

You see, thyroid disorders are often driven by a lack of adequate nutrients. Thyroid issues are also often made worse by trigger foods like gluten, dairy, and soy as described on page 153. And protein makes up the structure of hormones and makes up the structure of the thyroid gland. For this reason, the cornerstone of a diet for healing the thyroid is protein foods like fish, grass-fed meats, eggs, wild game, pasture-raised poultry and pork, and seafood. These foods also contain anti-inflammatory fats that support a healthy thyroid.

Other fats for a healthy thyroid can and should include virgin unrefined coconut oil, coconut milk, avocados, extra virgin olive oil, grass-fed ghee, and sprouted seeds and nuts. You should also eat healing fermented foods like sauerkraut, unsweetened kombucha, apple cider vinegar with the mother, kefir, goat cheese, and fermented cow's milk cheese and yogurt if you can tolerate dairy.

Healing herbs and plants that you can use to support a healthy thyroid are nettles, ginger, lemon, turmeric, Boswellia, and licorice root (DGL licorice to avoid high blood pressure).

Vegan protein foods, sadly, are often triggers for thyroid problems. For example, soy and thyroid don't make for good company. This is because soybeans can have a goitrogenic effect and can reduce T_4 absorption as well as reduce thyroid hormone action (see page 20). While this may be only true if you have an iodine deficiency, you should know that most people do have iodine deficiency these days. Other legumes are high in anti-nutrients that can cause problems for the thyroid gland too.

Other things that you can do to keep your thyroid healthy is to filter your water-this help remove chlorine and fluorine which are hard on the thyroid gland. Last and perhaps most importantly, make sure to identify food sensitivities to foods like gluten and dairy which contribute to autoimmune thyroid disease.[17] A trial elimination of gluten and dairy should be for at least 3-4 weeks. I suggest adding these back one by one. Only add one at a time back and add each one for a period of 4 days. Don't add combination foods like pizza back either. The best way to add gluten back, for example, is to add back a saltine cracker or a water cracker because bread or pizza is most likely going to contain dairy, soy, or both. For a healthy thyroid, also avoid or minimize processed seed oils, alcohol, and sugar, and get lots of antioxidant-rich vegetables and fruits. Bear in mind that you should cook cruciferous veggies if you have a thyroid disorder to reduce their **goitrogen** content.[18] This is because cruciferous vegetables are high in goitrogens if they are raw.

Chapter 6

Endometriosis

Endometriosis is **a** disease in which uterine tissue (endometrium) grows outside the uterus in areas like the pelvic organs, ovaries, Fallopian tubes, and surrounding abdominal tissues. If you don't have endometriosis, I'm guessing you know someone who does even if they don't talk about it much. Depending on the statistics you read, at least 10 percent of women struggle with endometriosis and 50 percent of women who are infertile have this painful condition.[19] Science has barely dipped its toe into the natural world and how it relates to endometriosis. If you try to find clinical studies about endometriosis in general they are few and far between. I'm willing to bet if such a painful condition afflicted men there would be stacks of research, but I digress.

You should know that putting this section together was a can of worms because there are little tidbits of research on many healing compounds but no consistent thread of any certain herb or food and barely any on conventional medications either. I took a further in-depth look at online forums and product reviews to help put together a more comprehensive list of healing compounds and plants here than what is strictly available in the Library of Medicine. This section was going to be short, but the further I dug in, the more complex this subject became. My goal is to give you or your loved one some tangible tools to help manage the pain and symptoms of this difficult and common condition.

Endometriosis and Inflammation

Endometriosis is absolutely related to what we put in our bodies because everything is. One common theme in research is that inflammation drives this condition.[20] If you have a genetic tendency to get endometriosis, the food and environment that your body is in cause the genes to pull the trigger on the progression to endometriosis. Everything is related to what we put in our bodies and can either drive more inflammation or dampen it.

Sadly, conventional anti-inflammatory therapies for endometriosis, such as ibuprofen, have bad long-term risks for the body and as mentioned earlier, result in altered estrogen metabolism. The end result of these anti-inflammatory medications isn't great. Other conventional therapies like Orlissa® can't be taken long term because they weaken the bones and cause liver problems.[21] In contrast, the intelligence of natural anti-inflammatory plants and foods benefits pain symptoms without the negative side effects in most cases. Progesterone also deserves attention especially if it is in the bioidentical form as discussed on page 140 and I will discuss how it relates to endometriosis on page 160.

For helping alleviate endometriosis, eating an unprocessed foods diet with lots of herbs and spices is going to be your best bet while avoiding food triggers.[22] There are some specific foods and herbs that are more likely to help or hurt than others. For many women, these triggers to avoid are gluten and dairy, but if you know something else upsets your gut, it's also causing inflammation in the body (yes your endometrial lining too), so the simple thing to do is avoid trigger foods. Let's take a deeper look at what is known and what isn't known about this debilitating condition.

Endometriosis and Diet: The Bad, The Good, and The Confused Scientists

> *Sugar and processed foods cause inflammation and are bad for every type of tissue, including the endometrium. This isn't negotiable and the research is clear on this topic; sugar is even related to an increased risk of endometrial cancer.*[23-26] *Cleaning up your diet with antioxidant-rich foods and minimizing sugar and processed foods is critical to minimizing symptoms of this condition.*

Gluten from most grains likely makes endometriosis pain worse for most women. One shining example of this is a naturalized study of a gluten-free diet on symptoms of endometriosis. It was published in an obscure journal and didn't get a lot of attention but it should have. This is because a striking 75% of women following a gluten-free diet for a year had a reduction in endometrial pain over the course of the year of a gluten-free diet.[27]

Larger studies aren't always better in the case of endometriosis risks. For example, one study about endometriosis suggested that higher vegetable intake increased the risk of endometriosis while gluten was associated with lower risk[28]. These types of population studies don't capture food intake well. This is because everyone in the world is told to eat gluten via "whole grains". Gluten is found in almost all junk foods. The study results were nonsensical based on hormones' actions in the body.

The first study I mentioned about a gluten-free diet means more because it showed a reduction in pain following a gluten-free diet for over a year. Research design matters and this was an active study and a long-term treatment. After all, it's impossible to fake endometriosis symptom reduction, or have a placebo effect, for a year. The larger study was fraught with poor design methods and no active treatment.

The inflammation and symptoms of endometriosis are complex, so the natural treatments you choose shouldn't be a one-stop shop either. Aim to tackle the inflammation of endometriosis through multiple avenues: through food, herbs, and nutrient supplements.

Here is an overview of the natural compounds from diet and supplements that help reduce endometrial symptoms:

Fish oil supplementation reduces endometrial pain[29]. Fish and fish oil supplements are great for reducing inflammation and as such, help reduce pain across almost every aspect of health and the body. Quality and quantity matter as does the amount of time you take it as reviewed on page 44.

Turmeric: Whether you decide to eat turmeric daily or supplement turmeric, it should be one you definitely consider. According to early research, turmeric has the fascinating ability to reduce the blood supply to endometrial tissue that grows outside the uterus but maintains the blood supply to the endometrial lining in the uterus.[30] It is a very effective anti-inflammatory plant that likely reduces the growth of endometrial cells outside of the uterus by decreasing harmful estrogen and through other anti-inflammatory actions.[31-32] It should be one you consider for sure. Some people don't tolerate turmeric, so a good alternative in these cases is Frankincense. Refer back to page 100 for the best ways to supplement turmeric.

Frankincense, also known as Boswellia, is one of the more promising natural remedies for endometriosis because it has anti-inflammatory compounds that reduce endometrial formation and adhesion in cell and tissue studies.[33] It works great for reducing joint pain too.[34] Doses of 1000 mg per day are often used and try to find supplements with 65% boswellic acids.

Natural B-Vitamins and Probiotics: Research shows that people with endometriosis often have low levels of B-vitamins.[35] Using a combination of B-vitamins (use only methylated natural forms, not synthetic ones like folic acid), I like Thorne and Pure Encapsulations B-Complex brands. Using B-vitamins and probiotics together is good because probiotics help the body produce and absorb more B-vitamins, especially probiotics that contain Lactobacillus Plantarum, Lactobacillus reuteri, Bifidobacterium adolescentis and other Bifidobacterium strains. A bonus to adding probiotics is that they help regulate hormones. Probiotics likely help people with endometriosis because gut dysbiosis is common in women with this condition.[36]

Licorice Root has powerful antioxidant effects and gut healing benefits. A lot of times it can replace stomach acid medications for heartburn too. In addition, licorice root works similarly to treatments like Orlissa® and ibuprofen for endometriosis according to animal studies and cell studies.[37-39] As a bonus, licorice doesn't have the negative effects on bone health, kidney health, and liver health that these drugs do. Just keep in mind that one possible side effect of licorice root is that it can increase blood pressure and lower blood potassium levels. To avoid these potential side effects, you can use the DGL form of licorice root. Typically, doses of around 300 mg of DGL licorice are used per day.

Ceylon Cinnamon as part of Traditional Chinese Medicine combinations (see herbal combination section on page 120) can be helpful for endometriosis and it makes sense because cinnamon generally helps reduce painful periods and associated inflammation with a high measure of safety. Be sure to use true cinnamon as Ceylon cinnamon.

Quercetin is a potent antioxidant that has the amazing ability to prevent the growth of endometrial tissue outside of the uterus, at least according to animal studies.[40-41] It is great for reducing inflammation and is natural with little to no risk of side effects if used in doses of 500-1000 mg per day. It has some side benefits too because it can help reduce allergy symptoms and help promote healthy immune function.

Zinc Supplements: Zinc deficiency is related to the development of endometrial growths outside of the uterus.[42] Adding to this, supplementing zinc helps reduce pain in women with **dysmenorrhea.**[43] While no studies have determined if zinc supplements help endometriosis, a deficiency of zinc likely makes endometriosis worse. Many medications also rob the body of this mineral. Women are frequently low in zinc because they often avoid zinc-rich foods-the media and the internet tell us to avoid these foods like beef and other meats.

Pine Bark helps with so many things as described in Chapter 5 and endometrial pain is one of those things. Doses used for endometriosis pain are 60 mg per day but give it at least 2 months to begin to work.[44]

Resveratrol is similar to pine bark in that it is a potent antioxidant but it is derived from grapes instead of pine. It is more expensive than pine bark but has some fascinating benefits for endometriosis. Doses of 30 mg per day of resveratrol have been given alongside hormonal therapy; adding resveratrol at this dose helps provide complete resolution of pelvic pain in 82% of women using it.[45] Not too shabby of results!

Zedoaria and Sparganium are two plants used together in Traditional Chinese Medicine to help aid in many period issues. Zedoaria is related to turmeric and ginger and Sparganium rhizome is used for painful periods and for helping women who have amenorrhea (don't get periods). Early research shows that it has bioactive compounds that antagonize estrogen and reduce the growth of cancer cells.[46] As such, these two compounds have been used effectively for many women. Using Traditional Chinese Medicine is always best under the guidance of trained herbalists.

Melatonin is best known for aiding sleep, but it does so much more. It is a natural antioxidant that is present in foods that helps aid in immune function. A small clinical study conducted over 8 weeks found that it reduces endometrial pain by almost 40%, reduces period pain by about the same amount, improves sleep quality, and helps normalize bowel function in women suffering from endometriosis.[46] Doses of 10 mg per day were used in this study.

Progesterone Progesterone Progesterone As mentioned previously, using natural progesterone derived from wild yam or using wild yam can be a godsend in endometriosis. Two-thirds of women with the condition respond very well to bioidentical progesterone with a major reduction in endometriosis symptoms.[48] Dosing of progesterone in this case should be fine-tuned with a trained practitioner who uses bioidentical progesterone. Some women experience progesterone resistance after treatment, but obtaining adequate vitamin A as retinol in the diet or in supplements from organ meats may help prevent this resistance.[49] So can eating an anti-inflammatory diet rich in whole foods as discussed in Chapter 3 and in the recipe and meal planning section.[50]

Vitex: It also makes sense to try Vitex which is an herb discussed in Chapter 5 in detail because it supports your own body's progesterone production and helps strengthen your body's resilience to most any women's issue. Vitex may also help endometriosis because it helps aid in a normal luteal phase in the menstrual cycle.[51]

Cramp Bark is basically self-descriptive in that it reduces cramps and some research shows that it may reduce adhesion of endometrial tissue.[52] Herbalists often recommend Cramp bark 300 mg three times daily, preferably enhanced by Ginger root, Rutin, Vitamin C, Vitamin E, Vitamin B3, Vitamin B6, and Magnesium citrate.

Feverfew is an anti-inflammatory herb sometimes referred to as Parthenium, that is in the daisy family of plants. Most research shows that feverfew is effective for pain conditions like migraines but is also effective for reducing allergy symptoms. Not much is truly known about how it may reduce endometrial pain, but it may do so by reducing inflammation and by easing muscle spasms.[53] Doses of 100-300 mg up to 4 times daily. Be aware that some people have a sensitivity to this plant and if this is you, please avoid using it.

Cannabis is a natural anti-inflammatory plant with well-known pain-relieving benefits. Many women find this herb to be the most beneficial for endometrial pain and it's hard to argue with that.

Red Raspberry Leaf is a great overall women's tonic and women often report that it helps reduce their endometrial issues. It's best to drink this tea daily or get a high-quality red raspberry leaf supplement as detailed on page 102.

Skullcap sounds scary but is related to mint and has a gorgeous purple flower on it. Not only does skullcap help with mood and reduce anxiety, this beneficial plant helps reduce the growth of endometrial cells in cell studies too.[54-55] However, this is one I recommend you take under the guidance of a reputable naturopath because there are some potential side effects, especially at higher doses.

Motherwort is also helpful for women with endometriosis, but only self-reports exist, sadly. No clinical trials are out there at this time. Luckily it's a safe herb to try as reviewed on page 116. It is also good for the heart and very calming in my experience.

Herbal Combinations: Online forums are sometimes helpful for managing endometriosis and in these, Traditional Chinese Medicine is often cited as helpful. Gui Zhi Fu Ling Wan is an herbal combination often suggested, but I would seek out the help of a trained herbalist before embarking on this type of treatment. This herbal combination contains cinnamon, peony, peach seed, and poria. Here is a review study of herbal remedies in Traditional Chinese Medicine Published in Evidenced-Based Medicine in Complementary and Alternative Medicine.

Other Supplement Combinations: One study used quercetin, turmeric as curcumin, feverfew, niacin (as nicotinamide), natural folate as 5-methyl etrahydrofolate, and omega 3 for endometriosis symptoms.[56] The people receiving this supplement regimen had much fewer endometriosis symptoms than those who didn't get the supplements. This study makes sense because folate metabolism is impaired in women with endometriosis. In other words, avoid synthetic folate called folic acid and choose natural folate sources from foods like leafy greens and eggs and natural folate supplements like 5-methylfolate or folinic acid.

Phytoestrogens: Friend or Enemy for Endometriosis?

Phytoestrogens have anti-inflammatory properties and hormone augmenting properties that may be useful in managing endometriosis[57]. Great choices of phytoestrogen foods and herbs are ashwagandha, red clover, resveratrol, pomegranate, green tea, oranges, celery, chamomile, milk thistle, artichoke, parsley, apples, fennel, cranberries, blueberries, passion flower, and believe it or not, honey. Chamomile holds a lot of promise because some of its other active compounds may be helpful for reducing endometrial cell growth.[58]

Soy foods like miso, tempeh, tofu, soy milk, and other fermented soy products like natto can be good choices for some women if and only if they are organic as outlined on page 48. However, you should know that endometriosis is most common in Asian women who tend to eat more soy[59]. In contrast, endometriosis rates are lowest in black and Hispanic women who tend to eat very little soy. But just like most things women-related, there is very little research devoted to this topic so it may or may not be a real variance between race and ethnicity due to under reporting in under-served populations. My hunch is that organic soy foods may help some women, but aren't going to be the complete answer or an answer for all. One way to know is to try to eat it consistently for a couple of months and see if your symptoms improve or worsen. But you should know that there are women out there that find that they feel worse with soy, so I'm making no promises. Honestly, if it were me, I would stick with the other phytoestrogens listed in the previous paragraph because they have complex anti-inflammatory compounds in other ways.

Polycystic Ovarian Syndrome (PCOS)

"PCOS may be part of my story, but it doesn't dictate the ending. "
  -Unkown

While PCOS affects women mostly that are overweight, many thin women bear the symptoms of this condition too because of all the toxic foods in our environment and insulin resistance doesn't discriminate based on weight. Almost one-third of women have PCOS and 40% have at least 2 symptoms of PCOS according to a study of students, faculty, and staff at Texas Woman's University.[60] This is simply an unacceptable rate of pain and illness amongst supposedly healthy women.

Common symptoms of PCOS are **ovarian cysts**, irregular periods, infertility, acne, excess facial hair, and a "beard" of acne because it tends to occur on the chin and jaw. But, acne can also be on the back with this condition.

Major websites, including the Mayo Clinic, present hormonal birth control as one of the main options to manage this condition.[61] Wow, really? Remember, on hormonal birth control women most often don't ovulate. PCOS is plagued by infertility, so how can a therapy that stops ovulation be among the best solutions? While the Mayo Clinic website does go on to suggest weight loss, they give no tangible ways to do so. And hormonal birth control and breast cancer treatment drugs they suggest do nothing to fix the underlying insulin resistance and create a whole new host of side effects. Alternatively, managing PCOS naturally gets to the root of the problem and doesn't just simply mask it. While I'm not saying that there isn't a time and a place for birth control, PCOS isn't fixed best by things coming from a pharmacy.

Looking back on the symptoms I had in my 20s, I'm sure I had some of the abnormal hormone patterns of PCOS, thyroid disorders, eating disorders, and heavy periods all wrapped up into one. My main PCOS symptoms were in how my acne appeared, heavy periods, and ovarian cysts. Once I cleaned up my diet, chose key herbal and dietary supplements, and eliminated food sensitivities, all my PCOS symptoms went away. This can happen for you too and I'll demonstrate how.

If you have PCOS, there is luckily more research behind this condition than most when it comes to abnormal periods. As discussed in most of the previous chapters, there are a lot of diet strategies and healing supplements that can help you be well on your way to recovery from this disorder.

As a refresher, PCOS is often driven by excess insulin as a result of insulin resistance, excess estrogen, excess testosterone, and too little progesterone. Another driver of PCOS is inflammation and because of this, the vast majority of remedies discussed in this book can help PCOS too.

Fixing the diet is the cornerstone here. By ditching processed carbohydrates, gentle intermittent fasting, and eating healing foods, you will be on your way to recovery from PCOS.

Quick Tip: Fasting Works Well for PCOS

While I haven't mentioned intermittent fasting much, you should know that it has a tremendous ability to help reduce PCOS symptoms. Sure, I hear every critic out there..."but the studies are small!" or "fasting is hard!" Correct, they are small, but no, fasting isn't hard at all and I'll explain how to do it so you won't feel deprived.

While yes, the studies done with fasting so far are small, a small study with a huge beneficial effect is still better than a large study with a small effect. And the beneficial effect size so far in the clinical trials where intermittent fasting is used is MAJOR[62]. In fact, simply eating over an 8-hour window throughout the day and fasting the other 16 hours in the day significantly reduced body weight, body fat, visceral fat (the BAD fat in your belly), testosterone, inflammation, glucose, and all the while improved insulin resistance in women with PCOS. Not only that, 73% of women had improved period cycle regularity with fasting alone.[62]

A ketogenic diet and fasting diets have a lot in common. Both help mobilize fat to burn as energy and help the bodies use ketones, a fuel the body uses when burning fat, as an energy source. A ketogenic diet and fasting both diminish insulin resistance too. Women following a ketogenic diet had similar improvements in all of these same markers of PCOS in a couple of research studies[63-64]. From a practical standpoint, however, intermittent fasting is a fair amount easier than a ketogenic diet to do for most women if they do it correctly.

Here is how you do it:

Starting fasting gradually and gently by eating over a 14 hour window in the day and fasting for 10 hours at night for the first week. Then in week two, increase your fasting window to 12 hours of fasting, 12 hours of eating throughout the day. By week 3, you can adapt to a schedule of 14 hours of fasting and 10 hours of eating. The other thing to remember is that you can be flexible with fasting and do it a few days of the week rather than all of the time. In my experience, though, the more you adapt to the fast, the less hungry you feel and the easier it is to do it. The most important piece to keep with the fast is to stay well hydrated and keep up on electrolytes. This simply means that you can add a pinch of Himalayan salt to the water you are drinking: when you fast you lose more sodium so don't worry about getting too much salt with a pinch of salt. If you want to try an electrolyte powder, this can work too but make sure it has at least 100 mg of salt in it.

Personally, I fast for 16 hours a day at least 4 days a week, but give myself a break from fasting when I need it by listening to my body about hunger. If the tank is too empty, I eat, plain and simple. Please listen to your body. But, as such, many people have been told their whole lives to graze on food all day and may be out of touch with true hunger because of this. That is why you should be gentle with yourself and give yourself grace. We all are different and if you can't find yourself doing this, seek out help from a person who is trained in intermittent fasting to help you along the way. I suggest checking out "The Diabetes Code" by Dr. Jason Fung because he is an honest physician with tons of helpful tips about how to fast successfully. Skipping fasting is during active menstruation is advised according to some evidence.-Sara Gotfried, MD "Women, Food, and Hormones."

Meal Plan and Supplement Strategies for PCOS

Beyond fasting, following a healing diet as described in the menu section of this book can help dampen inflammation and help normalize hormonal levels. Remember too, that if you are sensitive to any foods, it will throw off your hormone balance: I'm looking at you, gluten, dairy, and soy. See the section on Natural Thyroid Remedies on page 153 about how to properly eliminate these foods effectively and reintroduce them to determine food sensitivities.

Also, be mindful that raw broccoli or other cruciferous veggies help to normalize some of the toxic estrogen in the body related to PCOS and I suggest eating it at least every other day.

And in brief, a review of the supplements or culinary plants that can be helpful in this condition are vitamin D (please also check your blood levels and optimize them) and magnesium along with vitamin K2, milk thistle, black cumin seed, turmeric, quercetin, Vitex, coenzyme q10, ginkgo, tribulus, tulsi, wild yam cream, cinnamon, and especially inositol as reviewed in Chapters 4 and 5. Let's dive into more detail on some of these supplements and how they specifically help women with PCOS.

Inositol-women with PCOS taking inositol supplements were **almost twice as likely to have a normal menstrual cycle** as women who weren't using inositol in a study of women with PCOS as reviewed on page 74. Many women notice their PCOS acne disappears with inositol too. Doses of 4000 mg of myo inositol are often used while 300-600 mg of chiro inositol are effective.

Quercetin-improves insulin sensitivity as does milk thistle, cinnamon, turmeric, and black cumin seed. Using 1000 mg per day of quercetin is a common dose.

Tribulus-may help you by improving muscle-to-fat ratios in your body and just making you feel more human; it does for me. Remember that herbs and antioxidant-rich plants help the body reduce inflammation and help to detoxify hormones naturally, so getting a wide array of antioxidants through natural substances like tribulus, herbs, and spices in your diet is incredibly important for recovery from PCOS.

Herbal Combinations -I suggest trying a combination herbal blend like those found in Thorne SAT supplements which is a combination of milk thistle, artichoke, and turmeric. This combination helps insulin sensitivity while naturally dampening inflammation. You could certainly consider taking these herbs separately as well as described in Chapter 5.

Bioidentical Progesterone-as reviewed at the beginning of this chapter, is a topical supplement that should be considered for PCOS after discussing this with your naturopath or functional medicine provider. I have a friend with PCOS and her doctor told her that topical progesterone cream doesn't exist. It most definitely does, and it most definitely works. And even better, you can find it over the counter and this is a good option if your provider ignores your symptoms or they want to give you synthetic or oral progesterone only and you can't tolerate either. But I suggest finding a provider who is familiar with doses that are tailored for you.

Vitex-is another good option to help support normal progesterone levels but remember to be patient and give it at least a couple of months to become effective. Similarly, wild yam topical cream too is a good bet with no side effects. See chapter 5 to review its fascinating benefits. Doses of 750-1000 mg are commonly used in research.

Ceylon Cinnamon-in cooking, teas, and supplements also helps improve glucose levels and reduce insulin resistance so it can be helpful for women with PCOS.[65] Doses of up to 420 mg 3 times daily have been used for supplements of Ceylon cinnamon.

Magnesium-helps women who have PCOS because it reduces testosterone levels while increasing the hormone precursor called DHEA, the parent to progesterone and estrogen. It also helps decrease weight and increases luteinizing hormone, often a core hormone deficiency in women with PCOS.[66] The dose of magnesium used in this clinical trial was 250 mg per day.

Minimizing Uterine Fibroids The Natural Way

Uterine fibroids are benign growths in the uterus identified by ultrasound that can cause heavy bleeding and/or painful periods, AKA irregular periods, urinary frequency, constipation, belly pain and/or painful sex. Fun, huh?! The rate of uterine fibroids also has almost doubled from 1990 to 2019 indicating that foods and our environment are a major causal factor or at least contributing to the rise in cases. Almost 10 million women worldwide have this disabling and painful condition although they are almost certainly underdiagnosed.[67] I have had heavy periods my whole life and never have had an ultrasound offered for my heavy period issues with multiple providers over my life so I'm willing to bet that they are exceedingly underdiagnosed.

But, diagnosis sometimes is a can of worms because the conventional treatment options aren't awesome. Hysterectomies, hormones, other dangerous pharmaceuticals, repeat, no matter where you go. A hysterectomy is a major surgery and many women have lived to regret this decision. This isn't to say that there isn't a time and a place for these surgeries, but you should know that there are gentle things to try for these benign conditions before you go under the knife. And please, I beg you, vet out your surgeon carefully if you do go the hysterectomy route.

At the risk of sounding like a broken record, uterine fibroids are related to inflammation in the body, what we eat, and how we live our lives. But you should know that certain genetics also make these painful but benign tumors more likely. Even if you do have genetic risks for fibroids, there is so much you can do to prevent or lessen the risk of these and even help shrink them with diet and supplements.

Here are many examples of how you can help yourself. I suggest taking a multi-pronged approach and using several of the strategies next.

1. **Take vitamin D3 supplements** because they help shrink fibroids: One study showed that 50,000 IU vitamin D supplements every 2 weeks reduced the size of fibroids by a whole 10 millimeters over a period of 10 weeks. However, common sense supplementing is better given daily doses at smaller doses, such as 5,000 IU per day. But it's also smart to check your blood levels and add in more if you need it. Plus, vitamin D is good for balancing hormones in general.[68-69]
2. **Lower your insulin load**: Consider gentle intermittent fasting as

described in the Polycystic Ovarian Syndrome section on page 165 and avoiding sugar and processed foods because they spike insulin and IGF1. This is because insulin and IGF1 signal tissues like fibroids to grow, grow, grow. Herbs like milk thistle can be especially helpful because of this.[70]

3. **Bioidentical progesterone and/or wild yam creams:** can be a major benefit for reducing uterine fibroid symptoms.
4. **Avoiding plastics and endocrine disruptors:** like chemicals in foods as you should generally.
5. **Eat fish and/or take fish oil in its triglyceride form (cod liver oil):** because it reduces inflammation and fibroids thrive in inflammatory bodies.[71]
6. **Green tea extract:** may help shrink fibroids and help with fibroid symptoms. Research in this area used high doses of green tea at 800 mg per day.[72] For comparison, a cup of matcha green tea has about 57 mg of EGCG per 1 g of matcha green tea powder. To get the equivalent from tea would be 14 cups of matcha green tea. That's a lot of green tea and I don't recommend that. The green tea supplements are decaffeinated usually so they can actually be a good bet. You can start with a lower dose than the 800 mg per day and this would be my suggestion because higher doses can be nauseating and have some unwanted side effects.
7. **Turmeric:** is anti-inflammatory and may reduce fibroid growth. It is an essential for most hormonal conditions and has so many benefits for women with endometriosis. By decreasing inflammation, turmeric decreases the growth of uterine fibroid cells in early research.[73]
8. **Resveratrol or grape seed extract:** can help reduce inflammation and may help shrink fibroids.[74]
9. **Eat berries:** all kinds of berries provide ellagic acid, an antioxidant that may reduce fibroid growth. They also happen to be lower in sugar than most other fruits.
10. **Eat cruciferous veggies:** like broccoli, cabbage, Brussels sprouts, mustard, radishes, arugula, and watercress as described on page 40 because they reduce abnormal cell growth, neutralize estrogen, and

are anti-fibrotic too.

11. **Eat onions, garlic, chives, and shallots:** because they are anti-fibrotic in early studies.
12. **Lycopene foods:** help reduce fibrotic growth, reduce inflammation, and reduce abnormal cell growth. Great sources are tomatoes, watermelon, guava, papaya, grapefruit, and apricots.
13. **Ursolic acid foods:** including apple skin, marjoram, rosemary, oregano, sage, thyme, and peppermint have similar potential effects to the antioxidant foods listed here such as reducing fibrosis growth.[75] But be aware that these foods can have some drug interactions so make sure before you eat a bunch of them to check with your doc if you are on drugs like ACE inhibitors, ARBs for blood pressure, or cholesterol medications.
14. **Apigenin-rich foods:** similar to ursolic acid foods, apigenin foods have anti-fibrotic potential according to early research. These foods include chamomile, damiana, celery, parsley, artichokes, and oregano.[76]
15. **Quercetin:** naturally found in onions and apples, not only helps with PCOS, it may help prevent and treat fibroids. For more information about quercetin, see page 68. It has the opposite effect of estrogen on the uterus by reducing the chances of fibroid growth.[77]
16. **Avoid alcohol:** because it creates estrogen dominance and may fuel fibroid growth.
17. **Exercise regularly:** and in tune with your hormones as described on page 24 because exercise helps reduce stress hormones and reduces inflammation if done correctly.
18. **Iron supplements:** regardless of the cause of excess bleeding, iron deficiency is a result of excess bleeding, fibroids or not. Supplementing with iron is often a necessary and beneficial treatment because iron deficiency itself can cause, you guessed it, even more bleeding because it weakens the uterine wall.
19. **Most of the herbs in Chapter 5:** because herbs are intelligent plants that help naturally reduce inflammation and augment hormones gently.

20. **Vitex:** also known as chasteberry, is a popular natural remedy for PMS and hormonal balance. It has been suggested that vitex may help reduce uterine fibroids, although no specific studies show it can directly reduce the size of fibroids. However, its hormonal balancing effects may make it worth considering as a potential aid in managing fibroids.
21. **Manuka honey and propolis extract:** are rich in chrysin, which reduces estrogen and thereby may help reduce fibroid growth.[78]
22. **Magnesium supplements:** may help if you have been on long-term birth control or hormone replacement therapy. It also just generally helps promote well-being because it can help you sleep as reviewed on page 72.

Chapter 6 References

1. Whelan AM, Jurgens TM, Trinacty M. Bioidentical progesterone cream for menopause-related vasomotor symptoms: is it effective? Ann Pharmacother. 2013 Jan;47(1):112-6. https://pubmed.ncbi.nlm.nih.gov/23249728/
2. Ruiz AD, Daniels KR. The effectiveness of sublingual and topical compounded bioidentical hormone replacement therapy in post-menopausal women: an observational cohort study. Int J Pharm Compd. 2014 Jan-Feb;18(1):70-7. https://pubmed.ncbi.nlm.nih.gov/24881343/
3. Hermann AC, Nafziger AN, Victory J, Kulawy R, Rocci ML Jr, Bertino JS Jr. Over-the-counter progesterone cream produces significant drug exposure compared to a food and drug administration-approved oral progesterone product. J Clin Pharmacol. 2005 Jun;45(6):614-9. https://pubmed.ncbi.nlm.nih.gov/15901742/
4. Holtorf K. The bioidentical hormone debate: are bioidentical hormones (estradiol, estriol, and progesterone) safer or more efficacious

than commonly used synthetic versions in hormone replacement therapy? Postgrad Med. 2009 Jan;121(1):73-85. https://pubmed.ncbi.nlm.nih.gov/19179815/

5. Salem HF, Kharshoum RM, Abou-Taleb HA, AbouTaleb HA, AbouElhassan KM. Progesterone-loaded nanosized transethosomes for vaginal permeation enhancement: formulation, statistical optimization, and clinical evaluation in anovulatory polycystic ovary syndrome. J Liposome Res. 2019 Jun;29(2):183-194. https://pubmed.ncbi.nlm.nih.gov/30221566/

6. Livadas S, Boutzios G, Economou F, Alexandraki K, Xyrafis X, Christou M, Zerva A, Karachalios A, Tantalaki E, Diamanti-Kandarakis E. The effect of oral micronized progesterone on hormonal and metabolic parameters in anovulatory patients with polycystic ovary syndrome. Fertil Steril. 2010 Jun;94(1):242-6. https://pubmed.ncbi.nlm.nih.gov/19409554/

7. Holzer G, Riegler E, Hönigsmann H, Farokhnia S, Schmidt JB. Effects and side-effects of 2% progesterone cream on the skin of peri- and postmenopausal women: results from a double-blind, vehicle-controlled, randomized study. Br J Dermatol. 2005 Sep;153(3):626-34. https://pubmed.ncbi.nlm.nih.gov/16120154/

8. Abenhaim HA, Suissa S, Azoulay L, Spence AR, Czuzoj-Shulman N, Tulandi T. Menopausal Hormone Therapy Formulation and Breast Cancer Risk. Obstet Gynecol. 2022 Jun 1;139(6):1103-1110. https://pubmed.ncbi.nlm.nih.gov/35675607/

9. Stute, P., Wildt, L., & Neulen, J. (2018). The impact of micronized progesterone on breast cancer risk: a systematic review. *Climacteric*, *21*(2), 111–122. https://www.tandfonline.com/doi/full/10.1080/13697137.2017.1421925

10. Stephenson K, Neuenschwander PF, Kurdowska AK. The effects of compounded bioidentical transdermal hormone therapy on hemostatic, inflammatory, immune factors; cardiovascular biomarkers; quality-of-life measures; and health outcomes in perimenopausal and postmenopausal women. Int J Pharm Compd. 2013 Jan-Feb;17(1):74-

85. https://pubmed.ncbi.nlm.nih.gov/23627249/
11. Vigesaa KA, Downhour NP, Chui MA, Cappellini L, Musil JD, McCallian DJ. Efficacy and tolerability of compounded bioidentical hormone replacement therapy. Int J Pharm Compd. 2004 Jul-Aug;8(4):313-9. https://pubmed.ncbi.nlm.nih.gov/23924704/
12. Holtorf K. The bioidentical hormone debate: are bioidentical hormones (estradiol, estriol, and progesterone) safer or more efficacious than commonly used synthetic versions in hormone replacement therapy? Postgrad Med. 2009 Jan;121(1):73-85. https://pubmed.ncbi.nlm.nih.gov/19179815/
13. Dwivedi C, Heck WJ, Downie AA, Larroya S, Webb TE. Effect of calcium glucarate on beta-glucuronidase activity and glucarate content of certain vegetables and fruits. Biochem Med Metab Biol. 1990 Apr;43(2):83-92. https://pubmed.ncbi.nlm.nih.gov/2346674/
14. Ayyadurai VAS, Deonikar P, Fields C. Mechanistic Understanding of D-Glucaric Acid to Support Liver Detoxification Essential to Muscle Health Using a Computational Systems Biology Approach. Nutrients. 2023 Feb 1;15(3):733. https://pubmed.ncbi.nlm.nih.gov/36771439/
15. Dahlgren, M.K., Smith, R.T., Kosereisoglu, D. et al. A survey-based, quasi-experimental study assessing a high-cannabidiol suppository for menstrual-related pain and discomfort. npj Womens Health 2, 29 (2024). https://www.nature.com/articles/s44294-024-00032-0
16. Meditation Helps Eating Disorder Recovery. Greta Gleisner LCSW. https://www.psychologytoday.com/us/blog/hope-eating-disorder-recovery/201610/meditation-helps-eating-disorder-recovery
17. Should Your Thyroid Remedies Include a Gluten-Free Lifestyle? Thyroid Nutrition Educators. https://www.thyroidnutritioneducators.com/should-your-thyroid-remedies-include-a-gluten-free-lifestyle/
18. Best Food for Thyroid Patients. Thyroid Nutrition Educators. https://www.thyroidnutritioneducators.com/best-food-for-thyroid-patients/
19. Moradi Y, Shams-Beyranvand M, Khateri S, Gharahjeh S, Tehrani S,

Varse F, Tiyuri A, Najmi Z. A systematic review on the prevalence of endometriosis in women. Indian J Med Res. 2021 Mar;154(3):446-454. https://www.ncbi.nlm.nih.gov/pmc/articles/PMC9131783/
20. Khoufache K, Michaud N, Harir N, Kibangou Bondza P, Akoum A. Anomalies in the inflammatory response in endometriosis and possible consequences: a review. Minerva Endocrinol. 2012 Mar;37(1):75-92. https://pubmed.ncbi.nlm.nih.gov/22382616/
21. *Orilissa: Uses, dosage, side effects, warnings.* Drugs.com. (n.d.). https://www.drugs.com/orilissa.html
22. Sawalha K, Tripathi V, Alkhatib D, Alalawi L, Mahmood A, Alexander T. Our Hidden Enemy: Ultra-Processed Foods, Inflammation, and the Battle for Heart Health. Cureus. 2023 Oct 22;15(10):e47484. https://pubmed.ncbi.nlm.nih.gov/38022349/
23. King MG, Chandran U, Olson SH, Demissie K, Lu SE, Parekh N, Bandera EV. Consumption of sugary foods and drinks and risk of endometrial cancer. Cancer Causes Control. 2013 Jul;24(7):1427-36. doi: 10.1007/s10552-013-0222-0. Epub 2013 May 9. https://pubmed.ncbi.nlm.nih.gov/23657460/
24. Vennberg Karlsson J, Patel H, Premberg A. Experiences of health after dietary changes in endometriosis: a qualitative interview study. BMJ Open. 2020 Feb 25;10(2):e032321. https://www.ncbi.nlm.nih.gov/pmc/articles/PMC7044830/
25. Ilhan M, Güragaç Dereli FT, Akkol EK. Novel Drug Targets with Traditional Herbal Medicines for Overcoming Endometriosis. Curr Drug Deliv. 2019;16(5):386-399. https://www.ncbi.nlm.nih.gov/pmc/articles/PMC6637095/
26. Tassinari V, Smeriglio A, Stillittano V, Trombetta D, Zilli R, Tassinari R, Maranghi F, Frank G, Marcoccia D, Di Renzo L. Endometriosis Treatment: Role of Natural Polyphenols as Anti-Inflammatory Agents. Nutrients. 2023 Jun 30;15(13):2967.https://www.ncbi.nlm.nih.gov/pmc/articles/PMC10343861/
27. Marziali M, Venza M, Lazzaro S, Lazzaro A, Micossi C, Stolfi VM. Gluten-free diet: a new strategy for management of painful en-

dometriosis related symptoms? Minerva Chir. 2012 Dec;67(6):499-504. https://pubmed.ncbi.nlm.nih.gov/23334113/
28. Schwartz NRM, Afeiche MC, Terry KL, Farland LV, Chavarro JE, Missmer SA, Harris HR. Glycemic Index, Glycemic Load, Fiber, and Gluten Intake and Risk of Laparoscopically Confirmed Endometriosis in Premenopausal Women. J Nutr. 2022 Sep 6;152(9):2088-2096. https://pubmed.ncbi.nlm.nih.gov/35554558/
29. Nodler JL, DiVasta AD, Vitonis AF, Karevicius S, Malsch M, Sarda V, Fadayomi A, Harris HR, Missmer SA. Supplementation with vitamin D or ω-3 fatty acids in adolescent girls and young women with endometriosis (SAGE): a double-blind, randomized, placebo-controlled trial. Am J Clin Nutr. 2020 Jul 1;112(1):229-236. https://pubmed.ncbi.nlm.nih.gov/32453393/
30. Vallée, A.; Lecarpentier, Y. Curcumin and Endometriosis. *Int. J. Mol. Sci.* 2020, *21*, 2440.https://www.mdpi.com/1422-0067/21/7/2440
31. Zhang Y, Cao H, Yu Z, Peng HY, Zhang CJ. Curcumin inhibits endometriosis endometrial cells by reducing estradiol production. Iran J Reprod Med. 2013 May;11(5):415-22.https://www.ncbi.nlm.nih.gov/pmc/articles/PMC3941414/
32. O'Connell AA, Abdalla TE, Radulovich AA, Best JC, Wood EG. Curcumin Supplementation and Endometrial Lining: Examining the Role and Pathophysiology of Use During Frozen-Thawed Embryo Transfer. Cureus. 2021 Dec 14;13(12):e20415. https://www.ncbi.nlm.nih.gov/pmc/articles/PMC8754353/
33. Cho MK, Jin JS, Jo Y, Han JH, Shin S, Bae SJ, Ryu D, Joo J, Park JK, Ha KT. Frankincense ameliorates endometriosis via inducing apoptosis and reducing adhesion. Integr Med Res. 2023 Jun;12(2):100947.https://www.ncbi.nlm.nih.gov/pmc/articles/PMC10165193/
34. Bannuru, R. R., Osani, M. C., Al-Eid, F., & Wang, C. (2018). Efficacy of curcumin and Boswellia for knee osteoarthritis: Systematic review and meta-analysis. *Seminars in Arthritis and Rheumatism, 48*(3), 416–429. https://www.sciencedirect.com/science/article/abs/pii/S0049017218300027

35. Yalçın Bahat P, Ayhan I, Üreyen Özdemir E, İnceboz Ü, Oral E. Dietary supplements for treatment of endometriosis: A review. Acta Biomed. 2022 Mar 14;93(1):e2022159. https://www.ncbi.nlm.nih.gov/pmc/articles/PMC8972862/
36. Ata B, Yildiz S, Turkgeldi E, Brocal VP, Dinleyici EC, Moya A, Urman B. The Endobiota Study: Comparison of Vaginal, Cervical and Gut Microbiota Between Women with Stage 3/4 Endometriosis and Healthy Controls. Sci Rep. 2019 Feb 18;9(1):2204. https://www.ncbi.nlm.nih.gov/pmc/articles/PMC6379373/
37. Namavar Jahromi B, Farrokhnia F, Tanideh N, Vijayananda Kumar P, Parsanezhad ME, Alaee S. Comparing The Effects of Glycyrrhiza glabra Root Extract, A Cyclooxygenase-2 Inhibitor (Celecoxib) and A Gonadotropin-Releasing Hormone Analog (Diphereline) in A Rat Model of Endometriosis. Int J Fertil Steril. 2019 Apr;13(1):45-50. https://pubmed.ncbi.nlm.nih.gov/30644244/#
38. Wang XR, Hao HG, Chu L. Glycyrrhizin inhibits LPS-induced inflammatory mediator production in endometrial epithelial cells. Microb Pathog. 2017 Aug;109:110-113. https://pubmed.ncbi.nlm.nih.gov/28552807/
39. Namavar Jahromi B, Farrokhnia F, Tanideh N, Vijayananda Kumar P, Parsanezhad ME, Alaee S. Comparing The Effects of Glycyrrhiza glabra Root Extract, A Cyclooxygenase-2 Inhibitor (Celecoxib) and A Gonadotropin-Releasing Hormone Analog (Diphereline) in A Rat Model of Endometriosis. Int J Fertil Steril. 2019 Apr;13(1):45-50 https://www.ncbi.nlm.nih.gov/pmc/articles/PMC6334018/
40. Cao Y, Zhuang MF, Yang Y, Xie SW, Cui JG, Cao L, Zhang TT, Zhu Y. Preliminary study of quercetin affecting the hypothalamic-pituitary-gonadal axis on rat endometriosis model. Evid Based Complement Alternat Med. 2014;2014:781684.https://www.ncbi.nlm.nih.gov/pmc/articles/PMC4228827/
41. Chaichian S, Nikfar B, Arbabi Bidgoli S, Moazzami B. The Role of Quercetin for the Treatment of Endometriosis and Endometrial Cancer: A Comprehensive Review. Curr Med Chem. 2023 Oct 9.

https://pubmed.ncbi.nlm.nih.gov/37861023/

42. Onuma T, Mizutani T, Fujita Y, Ohgami N, Ohnuma S, Kato M, Yoshida Y. Zinc deficiency is associated with the development of ovarian endometrial cysts. Am J Cancer Res. 2023 Mar 15;13(3):1049-1066. https://www.ncbi.nlm.nih.gov/pmc/articles/PMC10077050/

43. Teimoori B, Ghasemi M, Hoseini ZS, Razavi M. The Efficacy of Zinc Administration in the Treatment of Primary Dysmenorrhea. Oman Med J. 2016 Mar;31(2):107-11. https://www.ncbi.nlm.nih.gov/pmc/articles/PMC4861396/

44. Kohama T, Herai K, Inoue M. Effect of French maritime pine bark extract on endometriosis as compared with leuprorelin acetate. J Reprod Med. 2007 Aug;52(8):703-8. https://pubmed.ncbi.nlm.nih.gov/17879831/

45. Maia H Jr, Haddad C, Pinheiro N, Casoy J. Advantages of the association of resveratrol with oral contraceptives for management of endometriosis-related pain. Int J Womens Health. 2012;4:543-9. https://www.ncbi.nlm.nih.gov/pmc/articles/PMC3474155/

46. Jia Jia, Xiang Li, Xueyang Ren, Xiaoyun Liu, Yu Wang, Ying Dong, Xiaoping Wang, Siqi Sun, Xiao Xu, Xiao Li, Ruolan Song, Jiamu Ma, Axiang Yu, Qiqi Fan, Jing Wei, Xin Yan, Xiuhuan Wang, Gaimei She,Sparganii Rhizoma: A review of traditional clinical application, processing, phytochemistry, pharmacology, and toxicity, Journal of Ethnopharmacology. 2021; 268: 113571. https://www.sciencedirect.com/science/article/abs/pii/S0378874120334590

47. Schwertner A, Conceição Dos Santos CC, Costa GD, Deitos A, de Souza A, de Souza IC, Torres IL, da Cunha Filho JS, Caumo W. Efficacy of melatonin in the treatment of endometriosis: a phase II, randomized, double-blind, placebo-controlled trial. Pain. 2013 Jun;154(6):874-81. https://pubmed.ncbi.nlm.nih.gov/23602498/

48. Schwertner A, Conceição Dos Santos CC, Costa GD, Deitos A, de Souza A, de Souza IC, Torres IL, da Cunha Filho JS, Caumo W. Efficacy of melatonin in the treatment of endometriosis: a phase II, randomized, double-blind, placebo-controlled trial. Pain. 2013 Jun;154(6):874-81.

https://www.ncbi.nlm.nih.gov/pmc/articles/PMC10138736/

49. Monastra G, De Grazia S, De Luca L, Vittorio S, Unfer V. Vitamin D: a steroid hormone with progesterone-like activity. Eur Rev Med Pharmacol Sci. 2018 Apr;22(8):2502-2512.https://pubmed.ncbi.nlm.nih.gov/29762856/

50. Donnez J, Dolmans MM. Endometriosis and Medical Therapy: From Progestogens to Progesterone Resistance to GnRH Antagonists: A Review. J Clin Med. 2021 Mar 5;10(5):1085. https://www.ncbi.nlm.nih.gov/pmc/articles/PMC7961981/

51. Milewicz A, Gejdel E, Sworen H, Sienkiewicz K, Jedrzejak J, Teucher T, Schmitz H. Vitex agnus castus-Extrakt zur Behandlung von Regeltempoanomalien infolge latenter Hyperprolaktinämie. Ergebnisse einer randomisierten Plazebo-kontrollierten Doppelblindstudie [Vitex agnus castus extract in the treatment of luteal phase defects due to latent hyperprolactinemia. Results of a randomized placebo-controlled double-blind study]. Arzneimittelforschung. 1993 Jul;43(7):752-6. German.https://pubmed.ncbi.nlm.nih.gov/8369008/

52. Saltan G, Süntar I, Ozbilgin S, Ilhan M, Demirel MA, Oz BE, Keleş H, Akkol EK. Viburnum opulus L.: A remedy for the treatment of endometriosis demonstrated by rat model of surgically-induced endometriosis. J Ethnopharmacol. 2016 Dec 4;193:450-455. https://pubmed.ncbi.nlm.nih.gov/27647013/

53. Pareek A, Suthar M, Rathore GS, Bansal V. Feverfew (Tanacetum parthenium L.): A systematic review. Pharmacogn Rev. 2011 Jan;5(9):103-10.https://www.ncbi.nlm.nih.gov/pmc/articles/PMC3210009/

54. Brock C, Whitehouse J, Tewfik I, Towell T. American Skullcap (Scutellaria lateriflora): a randomised, double-blind placebo-controlled crossover study of its effects on mood in healthy volunteers. Phytother Res. 2014 May;28(5):692-8. https://pubmed.ncbi.nlm.nih.gov/23878109/

55. Jin Z, Huang J, Zhu Z. Baicalein reduces endometriosis by suppressing the viability of human endometrial stromal cells through the nuclear

factor-κB pathway *in vitro*. Exp Ther Med. 2017 Oct;14(4):2992-2998. https://www.ncbi.nlm.nih.gov/pmc/articles/PMC5585734/
56. Signorile PG, Viceconte R, Baldi A. Novel dietary supplement association reduces symptoms in endometriosis patients. J Cell Physiol. 2018 Aug;233(8):5920-5925. https://pubmed.ncbi.nlm.nih.gov/29243819/
57. Bartiromo L, Schimberni M, Villanacci R, Ottolina J, Dolci C, Salmeri N, Viganò P, Candiani M. Endometriosis and Phytoestrogens: Friends or Foes? A Systematic Review. Nutrients. 2021 Jul 24;13(8):2532. https://www.ncbi.nlm.nih.gov/pmc/articles/PMC8398277
58. Ryu S, Bazer FW, Lim W, Song G. Chrysin leads to cell death in endometriosis by regulation of endoplasmic reticulum stress and cytosolic calcium level. J Cell Physiol. 2019 Mar;234(3):2480-2490.
59. Dai, Y., Li, X., Shi, J. et al. A review of the risk factors, genetics and treatment of endometriosis in Chinese women: a comparative update. *Reprod Health* 15, 82 (2018). https://reproductive-health-journal.biomedcentral.com/articles/10.1186/s12978-018-0506-7#
60. Rao, Manisha MSa; Broughton, K. Shane PhDb; LeMieux, Monique J. PhDb. Cross-sectional Study on the Knowledge and Prevalence of PCOS at a Multiethnic University. Progress in Preventive Medicine ():p e0028, June 2020. https://journals.lww.com/progprevmed/fulltext/2020/06000/cross_sectional_study_on_the_knowledge_and.1.aspx
61. Mayo Foundation for Medical Education and Research. (2022, September 8). *Polycystic ovary syndrome (PCOS)*. Mayo Clinic. https://www.mayoclinic.org/diseases-conditions/pcos/diagnosis-treatment/drc-20353443
62. Li C, Xing C, Zhang J, Zhao H, Shi W, He B. Eight-hour time-restricted feeding improves endocrine and metabolic profiles in women with anovulatory polycystic ovary syndrome. J Transl Med. 2021 Apr 13;19(1):148. https://pubmed.ncbi.nlm.nih.gov/33849562/
63. Paoli A, Mancin L, Giacona MC, Bianco A, Caprio M. Effects of a ketogenic diet in overweight women with polycystic ovary syndrome. J Transl Med. 2020 Feb 27;18(1):104. https://pubmed.ncbi.nlm.nih.gov/32103756/

64. Cincione RI, Losavio F, Ciolli F, Valenzano A, Cibelli G, Messina G, Polito R. Effects of Mixed of a Ketogenic Diet in Overweight and Obese Women with Polycystic Ovary Syndrome. Int J Environ Res Public Health. 2021 Nov 27;18(23):12490. https://pubmed.ncbi.nlm.nih.gov/34886216
65. Kort DH, Lobo RA. Preliminary evidence that cinnamon improves menstrual cyclicity in women with polycystic ovary syndrome: a randomized controlled trial. Am J Obstet Gynecol. 2014 Nov;211(5):487.e1-6. https://pubmed.ncbi.nlm.nih.gov/24813595/
66. Kort DH, Lobo RA. Preliminary evidence that cinnamon improves menstrual cyclicity in women with polycystic ovary syndrome: a randomized controlled trial. Am J Obstet Gynecol. 2014 Nov;211(5):487.e1-6.https://pubmed.ncbi.nlm.nih.gov/24813595/
67. Cheng LC, Li HY, Gong QQ, Huang CY, Zhang C, Yan JZ. Global, regional, and national burden of uterine fibroids in the last 30 years: Estimates from the 1990 to 2019 Global Burden of Disease Study. Front Med (Lausanne). 2022 Nov 7;9:1003605.https://www.ncbi.nlm.nih.gov/pmc/articles/PMC9676237/
68. Hajhashemi M, Ansari M, Haghollahi F, Eslami B. The effect of vitamin D supplementation on the size of uterine leiomyoma in women with vitamin D deficiency. Caspian J Intern Med. 2019 Spring;10(2):125-131. https://www.ncbi.nlm.nih.gov/pmc/articles/PMC6619469/
69. Islam, M. S., Akhtar, M. M., Ciavattini, A., Giannubilo, S. R., Protic, O., Janjusevic, M., Procopio, A. D., Segars, J. H., Castellucci, M., & Ciarmela, P. (2014, August). Use of dietary phytochemicals to target inflammation, fibrosis, proliferation, and angiogenesis in uterine tissues: Promising options for prevention and treatment of uterine fibroids?. Molecular nutrition & food research. https://www.ncbi.nlm.nih.gov/pmc/articles/PMC4152895/
70. Peiris AN, Sothmann MS, Aiman EJ, Kissebah AH. The relationship of insulin to sex hormone-binding globulin: role of adiposity. Fertil Steril. 1989 Jul;52(1):69-72. https://pubmed.ncbi.nlm.nih.gov/2663551/
71. Peiris AN, Sothmann MS, Aiman EJ, Kissebah AH. The relationship of

insulin to sex hormone-binding globulin: role of adiposity. Fertil Steril. 1989 Jul;52(1):69-72. https://pubmed.ncbi.nlm.nih.gov/26613601/

72. Peiris AN, Sothmann MS, Aiman EJ, Kissebah AH. The relationship of insulin to sex hormone-binding globulin: role of adiposity. Fertil Steril. 1989 Jul;52(1):69-72. https://www.ncbi.nlm.nih.gov/pmc/articles/PMC3742155/

73. Tsuiji K, Takeda T, Li B, Wakabayashi A, Kondo A, Kimura T, Yaegashi N. Inhibitory effect of curcumin on uterine leiomyoma cell proliferation. Gynecol Endocrinol. 2011 Jul;27(7):512-7. https://pubmed.ncbi.nlm.nih.gov/20672906/

74. Chen HY, Lin PH, Shih YH, Wang KL, Hong YH, Shieh TM, Huang TC, Hsia SM. Natural Antioxidant Resveratrol Suppresses Uterine Fibroid Cell Growth and Extracellular Matrix Formation In Vitro and In Vivo. Antioxidants (Basel). 2019 Apr 12;8(4):99. https://pubmed.ncbi.nlm.nih.gov/31013842/

75. Szydłowska I, Nawrocka-Rutkowska J, Brodowska A, Marciniak A, Starczewski A, Szczuko M. Dietary Natural Compounds and Vitamins as Potential Cofactors in Uterine Fibroids Growth and Development. Nutrients. 2022 Feb 9;14(4):734.https://pubmed.ncbi.nlm.nih.gov/35215384/

76. Melaibari M, Alkreathy HM, Esmat A, Rajeh NA, Shaik RA, Alghamdi AA, Ahmad A. Anti-Fibrotic Efficacy of Apigenin in a Mice Model of Carbon Tetrachloride-Induced Hepatic Fibrosis by Modulation of Oxidative Stress, Inflammation, and Fibrogenesis: A Preclinical Study. Biomedicines. 2023 May 2;11(5):1342.https://pubmed.ncbi.nlm.nih.gov/37239014/

77. Szydłowska I, Nawrocka-Rutkowska J, Brodowska A, Marciniak A, Starczewski A, Szczuko M. Dietary Natural Compounds and Vitamins as Potential Cofactors in Uterine Fibroids Growth and Development. Nutrients. 2022 Feb 9;14(4):734. https://pubmed.ncbi.nlm.nih.gov/35215384/

78. Balunas, M., Su, B., Brueggemeier, R., & Kinghorn, A. (2008). Natural products as aromatase inhibitors. *Anti-Cancer Agents in Medicinal*

Chemistry, 8(6), 646–682. https://www.ncbi.nlm.nih.gov/pmc/articles/PMC3074486/

Chapter 7

Empowering Your Life Phases

For this chapter, the natural phases of life will be explored and how you can help optimize how you feel. From PMS to menopause, learn some simple diet and supplement strategies to help you be your best version of yourself.

Premenstrual Syndrome (PMS)

This section requires no definition because the world jokes and complains so much about PMS that it bears no explanation.

If there ever was a thing that made women seem irrational and unstable, PMS is that thing. Sadly, this is such an unfair assessment of this cluster of symptoms women get during PMS and I'll tell you why. I also used to think PMS was something that needed to be conquered because it often feels so unnerving. But when I went to my clinical hypnotherapist, he explained that PMS is essentially the letting go of the feelings we held back and kept inside for the rest of the month that finally make their way out. Perhaps if we were better at asserting our needs and desires throughout the rest of the month, PMS would be more gentle on us. And it is, from what I have experienced.

Jokes and self-deprecating culture abound related to PMS and while it's nice to make light of situations if possible, the jokes take away our power and the beauty of shifts that comes with being a woman. And what I believe are intentional and necessary emotional and physical garbage that we kick to the curb when PMS comes around. Remember that even though men's mood swings often are as bad or worse than women's due to aggressive tendencies, there aren't any jokes about them. As women, we don't have to accept feeling lesser because of PMS: it's a powerful time in your cycle that promotes creativity and change, so try to harness it and above all, be gentle with yourself.

That said, PMS can make us feel out of control which isn't something that everyone is able to accept or want to accept. And there are some wild fluctuations in hormones that can make women feel rough, so there are some great strategies to make PMS feel more gentle and normal.

Eating a healthy diet should be a cornerstone of dealing with PMS. In fact, one of the few diet studies that exists about PMS and diet shows that junk foods that are high in sugar, processed fats, and salt are highly related to having more PMS symptoms.[1] On the opposite end, eating fruit is related to a reduction in PMS symptoms. But you should know that all other studies seem quite contradictory about diet and PMS. Still, remember that calcium-rich foods may help promote a sense of calm in the body and the mind, so including fermented dairy products like yogurt and cheese as well as calcium-rich sardines, almonds, seeds like sesame, and chia, and vegetables like broccoli, spinach, and kale can be part of a healthy mood solution for PMS.

Chapter 7

Foods to Eat for PMS

Even if there isn't a ton of research about how various foods affect PMS symptoms, you should know that nutrients are the building blocks of happy mood chemicals so without a doubt, what you eat affects the premenstrual experience. Regardless, you may still need to take some dietary supplements, but here is a chart of foods that may help keep PMS symptoms or any hormonal symptoms from starting in the first place.

The * symbol in this section indicates that gut imbalances or anti-nutrients in plant sources of these nutrients can impair absorption of these nutrients so supplements still may be needed to reduce PMS symptoms. You should also know that vitamin D from the sunlight is minimal if you use sunscreen or if you live in the northern hemisphere for most of the year.

- *Tryptophan: Turkey, crab, lamb, tuna, spirulina, pumpkin seeds, cheese
- *Tyrosine: Beef, organ meats, pork, chicken, fish, and organic tofu
- Vitamin A: Cod liver oil, beef liver, grass fed butter, egg yolks
- Vitamin C: Oranges, lemons, bell peppers, kiwi, rose hips
- *Vitamin D: Mid-day direct sunlight, oily fish, lard, cod liver oil
- *Vitamin B6: Organ meats, beef, fermented lentils, alfalfa, tuna, peas, bananas, cashews, turkey
- *Pantothenic Acid: Brewer's yeast, fermented brown rice, organic sunflower seeds, fermented organic corn, lentils
- *Vitamin E: Annatto, extra-virgin olive oil, spices, sunflower seeds, peanuts, broccoli, pecans, almonds
- *Calcium: Cheeses, bone broth, sesame seeds, kelp, broccoli sardines, bone-in canned salmon, almonds, Brazil nuts, watercress, dark green leafy vegetables, salmon, broccoli
- *Magnesium: Pumpkin seeds, beef, dark chocolate, sunflower seeds,

all nuts, oats, brown rice, dark green leafy vegetables, bananas, tuna.
- ***Zinc**: Oysters, beef, venison, clams, crab, chicken, cheese
- **Fatty Acids**: Cod liver oil, wild salmon, sardines, mackerel, egg yolks, borage, hemp seeds, black currant oil, evening primrose oil
- **Phosphatidylcholine and phosphatidic acid**: Broccoli and cabbage are particularly high in phosphatidic acid. Phosphatidylserine is found in organ meats, egg yolks, fish, and organic soybeans.

Did You Know...DHEA Can Help Perimenopause, Menopause, and Well Being

DHEA is a natural hormone originally derived from wild yams and is known as the fountain of youth. This may be because DHEA is the parent of the hormones estrogen, progesterone, and testosterone. As we age, our DHEA levels drop and this can contribute to symptoms of low libido and causes other hormones to be low. Low DHEA levels are also related to bone loss, aging signs, fatigue, low mood, and sexual dysfunction.[2] While this drop is a normal part of life for both men and women, some regions in the world sustain higher levels of DHEA despite age. I suspect this variance has to do with toxins, processed foods, and plastic use in certain regions. And low levels of DHEA are causal for a lot of hormonal issues that we have as women. Supplements of DHEA are protective for nerves, and improves mood and well-being for people over 40 years of age.[4-5] DHEA even helps reduce belly fat and improves insulin sensitivity in older women, so I'm a little surprised it isn't used more often[6]. Just make sure to check with your health provider before starting DHEA. Recommended doses are all over the map and can be as low as 2 mg per day and as high as 100 mg per day. Women tend to do better at doses around 10 mg or less as a starting dose. By the way, DHEA is also used to boost fertility in some settings in younger women. Using DHEA supplements is an amazing addition to my health routine and I can easily say it is one I won't live without because it helps my whole body feel younger, stronger, and more vital, including my sexual health.

Nutritional Supplements for PMS

Nutritional supplements have quite a bit of research behind them to show how they help with PMS symptoms. Here are some examples of how nutritional supplements may help your symptoms.

Vitamin B6-is quite helpful for reducing PMS symptoms and works even better when it is combined with magnesium supplements. Common doses of vitamin B6 are 40-50 mg and I highly suggest that you use the natural form called pyridoxal-5-phosphate or P5P. Magnesium supplements for PMS are usually dosed at around 250 mg per day.[7-9]

Vitamin D-is indispensable for all parts of our health and research shows it is also helpful for reducing PMS at high doses, 50,000 IU per week[10]. Vitamin D is better given daily dividing this dose up because of how it is used in the body, so a better schedule might be 5000-7000 IU per day, but have your blood levels checked. Low levels of calcium and vitamin D are both related to increased PMS symptoms during the luteal phase of menstruation.[11] This is the time when most women feel PMS symptoms.

5 HTP and Tyrosine-in my personal experience, are two amino acid supplements that are super beneficial for PMS symptoms and I take them together in a 10:1 ratio as recommended by many experts in the field, such as Dr. Amen. 5-HTP: 5-hydroxytryptophan (5-HTP), a form of tryptophan from foods, is the building block for happy mood chemicals in the body and brain called serotonin. 5-HTP is low in the brains of women with severe PMS called PMDD.[12] Additionally, low levels of tryptophan in the diet makes PMS worse[13]. Supplemental tryptophan helps reduce PMS symptoms[14]. It is often best to have 5-HTP along with L-tyrosine for many people because tyrosine helps to make the happy mood chemical called dopamine. [15-16] For more information you can read my blog all about L-tyrosine here: https://thehealthyrd.com/l-tyrosine-changed-my-life-and-it-may-change-yours-too/

Iron-is a nutrient involved in maintaining a healthy mood and memory.[17] Although no studies have directly looked at iron supplementation for PMS, using iron supplements luckily helps reduce heavy bleeding from menstruation as reviewed in Chapter 4. And as you may well know, heavy bleeding makes anyone feel tired and irritable the same as PMS does.

Vitamin E-is an antioxidant nutrient that helps provide PMS relief according to research.[18] Choosing natural vitamin E as mixed tocopherols or alpha tocopherol is the best option because synthetic vitamin E (dl-alpha tocopherol) can actually deplete the body of natural vitamin E.

Zinc-is an antioxidant mineral that may also help PMS by reducing symptoms of depression and improving quality of life with this condition.[19] However, like other nutrients, zinc supplements can take 3 months to help improve PMS symptoms. Zinc is worth your time no matter what because it is critical for immunity, brain health, and more. Just make sure to not exceed 50 mg per day in supplements as reviewed on page 70.

Fish oil-is rich in omega-3 fatty acids that reduce the severity of PMS according to a double-blind placebo controlled trial.[20] The longer that fish oil is used, the better it appears to work as well.[21] For added benefits of reducing heavy bleeding due to its vitamin A content, using cod liver oil should be considered instead of heavily processed fish oil supplements. Additionally, cod liver oil is better absorbed than most types of fish oil.

GLA-gamma linoleic acid helps reduce inflammation and PMS symptoms. It is found in evening primrose oil, borage oil, spirulina, and hemp seeds. Doses used in studies are typically between 180-500 mg per day. GLA reduces PMS severity and duration and reduces breast pain known as **mastalgia**.[22]

Probiotics-help balance hormones, so it is no big surprise that they also ease PMS symptoms.[23] They may even help reduce the severe version of PMS called PMDD. Research shows that probiotics are often very beneficial for anxiety and mood.[24] If you don't eat fermented foods like yogurt, cheese, and fermented vegetables, make sure to include a high quality probiotic supplement as described on page 41.

Oxaloacetate-a fascinating and safe supplement that is a natural form of energy produced in the body. This compound helps to support adequate glucose levels in the brain. Needs for energy in the brain during PMS go up, but unfortunately, eating sugar can worsen PMS symptoms. Supplemental oxaloacetate at 200 mg per day along with 300 mg of vitamin C reduces PMS symptoms according to one clinical study.[25] In fact, it reduces mood symptoms quite dramaticall. Reward: depression was reduced by 54% stress by generalized anxiety by 51%, and agression symptoms 18% and fascinatingly, suicidal thoughts by 48% too. While nothing works for everyone, if you suffer from severe PMS, I suggest giving oxaloacetate a try.

Phosphatidylserine & phosphatidic acid: are important structural parts of cell membranes which means they help hormones and nerve chemicals communicate from cell to cell more effectively. Supplements of 400 mg of each reduced symptoms of PMS in one study.[26] Interestingly, there was a significant reduction in the interference of PMS in relationships with others, 50% less anxiety, and increased productivity with this combination supplement. It also helped prevent elevations in the stress hormone cortisol.

Herbs for PMS Balance

Most of the herbs discussed in detail in Chapter 5 are beneficial for reducing PMS symptoms. Some of those that help to improve mood, bloating, and sleep disturbances during PMS include:

- **Saffron** helps improve mood across the board and is helpful in PMS similar to antidepressant prescriptions without the side effects.[27]
- **Vitex** reduces symptoms of PMS, such as headache, anger, irritability, depression, breast fullness, and bloating in multiple studies.[28-30]
- **Black Cohosh** doses of around 40 mg per day are effective for helping reduce hot flashes and its traditional uses for PMS benefit from similar dosing.
- **Turmeric**-reduces PMS by 50% according to research.[31]
- **Valerian Root** is very calming and promotes healthy sleep at doses of around 500 mg twice daily.
- **Ginger** is great for overall health and reduces mood swings during the premenstrual phase.[32]
- **St. John's Wort** promotes a happy mood during the luteal phase of menstruation. Just be careful to not use it if you are already on an SSRI medication.
- **Passion Flower** is overall calming and promotes a feeling of well-being.
- **Ginkgo Biloba** two studies show that ginkgo biloba also reduces PMS symptoms, especially breast tenderness.[33-34]
- **Dong Quai** is used traditionally for PMS and is often in PMS herbal blends.
- **Dandelion root** acts as a natural diuretic and is great to have as a tea or in doses described on page 117.
- **Damiana** is relaxing and I find it to be a perfect way to dampen down any rough mood edges. More research is needed but this herbal tea may help dampen the stress associated with PMS and help protect nerves[35]. It also is rich in antioxidants.[36]

- **Cannabis** helps reduce pain and also decreases anxiety symptoms, especially if you choose a strain of cannabis geared towards this[37]. Many people find broad-spectrum CBD or a 1:1 CBD to THC supplements is a helpful way to help manage PMS without the risks of over-the-counter pain relievers like ibuprofen. Just be sure to start with a low dose such as a few drops of tincture.

Beyond the ones mentioned in Chapter 5, here are some more herbs that you can try for getting a handle on your PMS symptoms.

- **Chamomile** is very beneficial for relaxation, improved sleep, and studies show that it reduces anxiety and water retention during PMS.[38]
- **Lavender** reduces PMS symptoms by enhancing **parasympathetic** activity of the nervous system and most research suggests that using oral lavender capsules works the best for relieving anxiety symptoms.[39-40]
- **Fennel** is healthy for the gut, which may be why it helps some people deal with PMS symptoms. It has antispasmodic effects which may also help with PMS symptoms[36]. It also helps hormonal balance overall according to research.[41-42]

Perimenopause

I crack myself up because the section I avoided writing about is the one that I'm most immediately facing: perimenopause. Somehow this phase of my reproductive life crept up on me and it has left me pondering, so much so, this section of the book stayed blank for a long time.

I was also procrastinating writing this because there is almost zero research and zero understanding of this mysterious phase our bodies go through. Unlike other period irregularities, perimenopause is a natural shift in hormones that is exceedingly unpredictable. This means you don't know what you are going to get on any given day.

Women in the perimenopausal stages face heavy periods, light periods, frequent periods, infrequent periods, debilitating pain, migraines, poor sleep, sore breasts, and lack of libido to name a few of the symptoms we can go through.

At the time I am writing this, there are around 6200 total publications on the subject in the Library of Medicine.[44] That may sound like a lot but it isn't because most of them just reiterate what other researchers say. Most of these perimenopause studies examine the levels of depression only and aren't proposing any interventions aside from synthetic hormones and pharmaceutical antidepressants. In contrast, there are around 30,000 publications about erectile dysfunction and 9,000 publications on Viagra ALONE.[45] This isn't even counting the 5 other erectile dysfunction drugs out there!

No one knows how long perimenopause will last for you. No one knows how bad it will be for you. Super helpful, right? Sometimes women have a lessening of their period symptoms but sometimes worsening overall during perimenopause. As such, your underlying root causes of hormonal issues should be addressed, such as insulin resistance, fibroids, endometriosis, PCOS, etc. At the root of most of these conditions is often too much insulin, inflammation, imbalanced thyroid, imbalanced cortisol, and too little progesterone. But I still think it's a good idea to check your baseline progesterone and follow-up hormone levels. Ask your provider to order these so you have something to work with.

But, a big word of caution; if you have unrelenting bleeding or very frequent bleeding, please do consult your doctor for appropriate workup. This can be a sign of uterine cancer, so don't avoid your doctor's visit and seek medical help.

On a lighter note, I have to tell you a silly story. My daughter is always coming up with funny phrases to add levity to serious things. She is such a joy. As my daughter and I were talking about perimenopause a while back, she coined perimenopause as "hairy many paws" because we both love cats, and likewise we should love this phase of life. But it also is aptly joked about because "hairy many pause" is a good way to describe the situation!

In regard to hormones during perimenopause, here are what the "experts" are saying; it lasts on average 5 years, and "The perimenopause is thus a time of cycle and hormone variability and single hormone measurements provide little useful information, with the clinical history being the most appropriate method of assessing menopausal status."[41]

The "experts" go on to say that "Estrogen will not reliably suppress perimenopausal estrogen levels; no clinical data have shown that hormonal therapy is effective or safe for perimenopausal **vasomotor symptoms**". In the same paragraph they go on to say "Yet, night sweats and sleep problems are major concerns among people in perimenopause, often starting when cycles are still regular and should be appropriately treated (with hormone replacement therapy)." This advice has no logic to it at all. They say giving synthetic estrogen doesn't work, but it is a good idea to do it anyway. The absurdity that surrounds women's healthcare is mind-blowing.

Seems like a whole lot of nonsense and a cop-out. I wish the world thought more broadly and deeply because women for thousands of years have known better by using herbal therapy and nutritional approaches to balancing hormonal fluctuations. These herbs and nutritious foods have anti-cancer and anti-inflammatory properties that reduce the risk of all chronic diseases too. Luckily, we still have some research that validates symptom management of perimenopausal symptoms using the gifts that the earth has given us. There really are a ton of options. Understanding the fundamental things that throw hormones off as discussed throughout this book are the things to keep in mind if you are in the perimenopausal phase.

Remember:

- Having more nutrients helps
- Reducing stress helps reduce cortisol
- Gentle exercise helps (but listen to your body)
- Progesterone often helps
- Herbs help
- High-quality sleep helps

Personally, adopting a solid regimen of herbal therapies including topical wild yam cream and topical progesterone cream along with organ meats and consistently taking my iron and cod liver oil have been exceptionally beneficial for me. I dare say that this phase of my life has become my favorite phase of life because I have taken my health back using natural approaches. Saffron, turmeric, black cumin seed oil, vitex, damiana, cannabis, and raspberry leaf tea are my best friends. And yes, there is surprisingly research about cannabis and how it helps women in perimenopause, especially in terms of mood swings.[47]

Bioidentical progesterone may be a great option for you and research shows that using 300 mg per day at bedtime is effective.[47] But again, do check in with your provider, and while progesterone helps, it can take some fine-tuning of when and how to take it. The body does naturally decline in hormones for a reason, so getting to the core of why you are making relatively too little progesterone, such as stress, lack of nutrients, and lack of healing herbs should accompany your journey through menopause.

Perimenopause isn't all bad; it's actually quite a good phase of life if you ask me. There can be a big advantage that I'm finding in perimenopause too over other phases I've been through. The mood swings of PMS are next to gone and I attribute this improvement in mood to my herbal regimen and diet regimen.

My Personal Story of Perimenopause Havoc

Bleeding is my uterus's default. As such, my uterus was having a grand old time bleeding every other week and the bleeding was HEAVY at one point during my perimenopause phase. While I was already implementing a lot of healthy strategies, I was under a lot of stress and admittedly, fell off some of my healthy habits for a few weeks like cod liver oil, iron supplements, and organ meats. One evening, as my period kicked in again after 3 in a row in one month, I felt desperate and so depleted that I had my husband take me to our health food store. Knowing that progesterone and wild yam might be helpful, I grabbed both topical creams and I also saw the Solaray Stages Perimenopause supplement and started taking it. I'm not joking; within an hour or two, the bleeding subsided, and by the next day was almost gone completely. By day two of using the two natural hormone creams, I stopped bleeding altogether. I should also mention that I never stop bleeding after two days. Even if it is a light period, it goes on for at least 5 days. So I fully attribute my normalization of periods to the wild yam and progesterone cream along with the perimenopause supplement. You know, the things that Google and your healthcare provider might tell you doesn't work? Or doesn't even know exists? Since then, I've enjoyed what I refer to as "normal girl periods" every 28 days that are moderate and pretty painless. I should also mention my use of motherwort because it helps reduce abnormal heart beats during this phase of my life and it works pretty quickly for this. While I'm back on my normal supplement routine again along with the wild yam and progesterone, I am delighted and feel balanced again. I can exercise without being wiped out; I kicked heavy bleeding to the curb and other perimenopausal symptoms by using what nature gave me. I took back my health without the need for factory-made pharmaceuticals. I discontinued the Solaray Perimenopause supplement because I found it too stimulating for me and instead just take black cohosh now. In addition, with the help of my naturopath and the DUTCH hormone test, I started taking DHEA supplements and this has helped me feel normal again along with my herbal concoctions.

The Nuts and Bolts of Supplements for Perimenopause

Here is an overview of the herbal and diet strategies for perimenopause that are discussed more fully in Chapter 3 and 4. I suggest trying one or more of the following remedies depending on the symptoms you may be having. Remember, herbs and supplements help, but they don't often help instantly so give them some time to do their work. While little research is devoted to the perimenopausal years, it doesn't mean that some of the therapies that work to balance stress hormones and progesterone won't also help you because I know from personal experience that they can and will if you combine them with a healthy diet and manage your stress.

- **Vitamins and minerals**: vitamin A and iron to reduce bleeding, vitamin D as a master hormone regulator, vitamin B6 as P5P for mood benefits, and an all-around natural B complex.
- **Balancing foods**: organ meats like beef liver, broccoli family vegetables to detoxify estrogen, getting plenty of protein (at least 0.7 grams per pound of your body weight per day), cooking with spices, herbs, and plenty of healthy fats, antioxidant-rich foods like berries, oranges, lemons, tea, root vegetables, and ditching junk foods if possible. See the meal planning and recipes section in Chapter 8 for more details.
- **To help reduce bleeding and pain**: bioidentical progesterone cream

and wild yam cream, vitex, turmeric, ginger, frankincense (Boswellia), dong quai, herbal blends like Solaray Stages, Vitanica Women's Phase 1 and 2.
- **Increase sexual function and urinary health**: resveratrol, ashwagandha, pine bark extract, nettles, and damiana tea.
- **Improve memory**: ashwagandha and ginkgo biloba.
- **Improve mood:** eating more high-quality protein and fats as reviewed on page 43, saffron, herbal blends like Solaray Stages, stress B complex in natural forms, cannabis, St. John's wort, betaine, vitex, bioidentical hormone creams, L-tryptophan (5-HTP) and L-tyrosine, SAMe.
- **For improving sleep:** magnesium supplements, natural vitamin B6 as P5P, cannabis (full-spectrum 1:1 THC: CBD ratio), damiana tea, chamomile tea/supplements, lavender tea/supplements, valerian root, passion flower, dong quai, and melatonin.
- **For reducing hot flashes and night sweats**: sage, black cohosh, St. John's wort, wild yam, dong quai, valerian root, and nettles.
- **For heart palpitations**: after you check with your doctor first, you can try adding motherwort which I find exceptionally helpful for calming down irregular heartbeats due to perimenopausal fluctuations.

Menopause

Just so we are all on the same page, menopause is the phase of life where periods have come to an end for good. If you have had period issues, which I assume you have because you are reading this book, this section is probably a time for celebration! Just like you can't exactly escape perimenopause, the phase of menopause is another part of life that people either anticipate with joy or dread because of the changes in their bodies that are separate from your period altogether.

It is possible to ease into menopause without unwanted effects, but it's not the usual. Across the world, women experience menopausal symptoms at varying degrees. Denmark, Norway, and Sweden have the lowest rates of complaints of menopause compared to the highest rates in the United States, Canada, and the United Kingdom. Of note, the countries with the lowest rates of complaints have the highest rates of preventive care. In Singapore, about half of women report menopausal symptoms while almost 85-90% of women experience them in India and the United States.[49-51]

Singapore also has a high rate of use of natural medicine use. I'm not saying this is why they have fewer menopausal symptoms than other regions but there could definitely be a connection made.[52-54]

The United States and India have exceedingly high rates of diabetes whereas Singapore does not. This connection is possibly why hot flashes are so common here. In fact, women with insulin resistance are much more likely to have hot flashes than those who do not. A high fasting insulin level predicts hot flashes. This goes back to the idea that too much carbohydrate intake and not enough time in the fasting period of your day may increase your risk of menopausal symptoms altogether.[55]

Hot flashes, also known as vasomotor symptoms, are the most commonly reported symptom of menopause. These vasomotor symptoms are both day and night-time episodic flushing and sweating. Some research shows that these flushing symptoms can be due to an abnormal cortisol awakening response and high daytime cortisol levels rather than anything to do with estrogen decline. Hot flashes, not surprisingly, are linked to higher inflammation levels in the body.[56-57]

And you shouldn't ignore hot flashes because they are linked to an increased risk of heart disease.

Blunted cortisol levels in the morning are a problem because they are related to heart palpitations too and the more severe the vasomotor symptoms you have, the higher your risk for heart disease is as well.[58]

Diet Tips for Menopause

By now you are probably connecting the dots with the fact that natural remedies can work better than conventional remedies for hot flashes because they often tackle all angles for balance in the body related to cortisol, estrogen, progesterone, and inflammation.

Cooking with the herbs and spices mentioned so far in this book can be so beneficial as can supplementing them if you aren't into eating them. These work to decrease daytime cortisol and also dampen inflammation, both of which are at the root of menopausal symptoms like hot flashes.

Eating a diet rich in collagen to support joint health and bone health as well as gut health is a good idea too. These foods include: organ meats, seafood, sardines, bone broth, chicken, pork, lamb, and grassfed beef. You can also find high-quality collagen powders on the market too. Cruciferous vegetables are natural estrogen stabilizers and cancer-fighting foods. Additionally, the phytoestrogen-rich foods, herbs, and spices listed on page 162 of the Endometriosis section such as chamomile, milk thistle, pomegranate, celery, and ashwagandha can be super helpful for menopause symptoms because they tackle the root causes of menopausal problems.

Did You Know....Black Cohosh to the Menopause Rescue

> It's definitely worth mentioning that black cohosh might be your next best friend if you are experiencing hot flashes and night sweats. At 8 weeks of use, of black cohosh, women had dramatic reductions, almost

75% less, in hot flashes according to a study. But you should know you need to give it at least 8 weeks to do its work. Studies that were shorter in duration didn't see the same benefits. This benefit magnitude is on par with hormone replacement therapy without any of the side effects.[59-60] A dose of 6.5 mg of black cohosh dry root extract was given in this study.

Also, you should know that black cohosh is rich in antioxidants which reduce inflammation levels, so this is likely the mechanism through which black cohosh works to reduce hot flashes. As a bonus, black cohosh helps boost mood and we all can use a bit of that in our lives!

Licorice Root for Cooling Effects

The one herb that is notorious for helping balance cortisol levels that first came to mind for me is licorice root. Not surprisingly, when I looked at the Library of Medicine, a study came up right away about how licorice root decreases hot flashes. So, it's not a big surprise then, that more so than estrogen, cortisol, and inflammation are the culprit when it comes to hot flashes. In this double-blinded, placebo-controlled trial, licorice root significantly reduced severe hot flashes and moderate hot flashes compared to placebo.[61] The group received 3 capsules daily containing 330 mg of licorice root. Just be aware that licorice root over time can increase blood pressure levels and lower potassium levels. You can use DGL type of licorice to avoid these risks.

Other Herbs That Reduce Hot Flashes

Beyond black cohosh and licorice root, here are some herbs and supplements, as discussed in Chapter 4 and 5, that can help reduce hot flashes and vasomotor symptoms. Refer back to this chapter for dosing and how to use them effectively.

- Sage
- Wild yam
- Valerian root
- Milk thistle
- Dong Quai
- Maca
- St John's wort
- Evening primrose oil

Other Herbs That Improve Sexual Function

There is a common theme in menopause: vaginal dryness and reduced sexual function. To help offset some of these symptoms, you should consider checking your hormones with the DUTCH test and have your provider correct any imbalances. In addition, the following herbs have traditional validation along with clinical studies showing their effectiveness for sexual function.

- Ashwagandha
- Ginkgo biloba
- Nettles
- Tribulus
- Maca
- Pine bark extract
- DHEA (from wild yam)
- Herbal blends as discussed on page 119

Herbs That Improve Energy and Memory

When going through menopause, you don't have to suffer from the reduced energy symptoms and memory complaints that many women have. Growing old gracefully can and should be within your grasp by using the time-honored and clinically-researched herbs here. Refer back to Chapter 5 for more information about how to use these herbs in your diet and in supplements.

- Sage
- Milk thistle
- Turmeric
- Ginkgo biloba
- Motherwort
- Maca
- Lions mane mushrooms

Herbs That Improve Mood

Just as is the case for PMS, herbs can help get you through mood changes that can occur with menopause.

These herbs are:

- Saffron
- Black cohosh
- St John's wort
- Tulsi
- Passion flower
- Motherwort

Chapter 7

Herbs That Decrease Inflammation During Menopause

Last but not least, eating an anti-inflammatory diet and using herbal remedies can go a long way to reducing the inflammation-related issues of menopause. In addition to all of the herbs listed in this menopause section, here are a few more to pay close attention to if you are suffering from symptoms of menopause.

- **Turmeric** helps reduce hot flashes quite significantly according to a clinical study of postmenopausal women. They used 500 mg of turmeric daily in this study[62].
- **Black cumin seed** helps improve blood glucose and blood fat levels in menopausal women when they receive 1 gram of black cumin seed per day.
- **Boswellia** may help get you to your physical activity goals because it reduces arthritis pain naturally.[63]

Cannabis is an antioxidant-rich plant that serves to dampen inflammation and even reduces colitis symptoms according to some studies. According to a Washington Post feature, many women who turn to cannabis to reduce their menopausal symptoms find it beneficial.[64]

Menstrual Migraines: Are Natural Remedies Better Than Conventional Treatment?

> Women who struggle with migraines during their menstrual cycles are rarely given options for helping their symptoms naturally. I've known many women who are only offered prescription medications for migraine treatment and these all come with a price to their health. But you should also know that migraines are often an outright sign of nutritional deficiencies. This can include magnesium deficiency, Vitamin B2, B6, and B12 deficiency, carnitine deficiency, and others.[65-68] Women who eat more omega-3 fats from fish while

limiting processed meats and aged cheeses (tyramine) and alcohol tend to also feel better if they have migraines.

Beyond these nutrients and food strategies, a safe antioxidant called coenzyme Q10 impressively reduces the severity, duration, and frequency of migraine headaches at doses as low as 100 mg per day.[69] This speaks to one of the major root causes of migraines; a lack of antioxidant balance.

It turns out that there are a whole host of other safe and natural herbs that help reduce migraines and also get to the root cause of these debilitating headaches. They do so by naturally dampening down inflammation and creating balance in the body and mind. One such example is butterbur, which is an herb with a great safety profile that reduces migraine frequency by almost 50% when taking 75 mg of it twice daily.[70] Feverfew, as reviewed on page 161, is another great option as a systematic review of 6 studies concluded that it is safe and effective for helping reduce migraine symptoms.[71] Vitex is a great option because it naturally increases progesterone, and research shows that progesterone is likely helpful for reducing migraine symptoms.[72] Another great remedy for migraines is pine bark extract, which is effective for many kinds of pain; the doses used in studies for migraines is 120 mg pine bark daily.[73]

If you have menstrual migraines, the best bet is to first tackle the condition nutritionally by using a high-quality B vitamin supplement as described on page 70, magnesium, and coenzyme Q10 100 mg per day. Doses of 400-600 mg of magnesium are effective and I suggest getting magnesium in powder or capsule form, not tablet form, for improved absorption[74]. Magnesium glycinate is the most readily available and best form of magnesium for migraines. L-carnitine is also a very safe option if these strategies don't work and it has no known toxicity. I wrote an extensive blog about L-carnitine if you want to check it out here: https://thehealthyrd.com/best-l-carnitine-supplement-brands-powerful-benefits/

As a quick fix, using intranasal peppermint at 1.5% concentration reduces severity of migraines quite quickly for many people.[75] Lavender aromatherapy is also a great option for reducing migraine according to many women. Just keep in mind that tackling the root causes nutritionally should be the cornerstone of migraine treatment and not a last resort.

Chapter 7 References

1. Hashim MS, Obaideen AA, Jahrami HA, Radwan H, Hamad HJ, Owais AA, Alardah LG, Qiblawi S, Al-Yateem N, Faris MAE. Premenstrual Syndrome Is Associated with Dietary and Lifestyle Behaviors among University Students: A Cross-Sectional Study from Sharjah, UAE. Nutrients. 2019 Aug 17;11(8):1939. https://www.ncbi.nlm.nih.gov/pmc/articles/PMC6723319/
2. Rabijewski M, Papierska L, Binkowska M, Maksym R, Jankowska K, Skrzypulec-Plinta W, Zgliczynski W. Supplementation of dehydroepi androsterone (DHEA) in pre- and postmenopausal women - position statement of expert panel of Polish Menopause and Andropause Society. Ginekol Pol. 2020;91(9):554-562. https://pubmed.ncbi.nlm.nih.gov/33030737/
3. Pluchino N, Ninni F, Stomati M, Freschi L, Casarosa E, Valentino V, Luisi S, Genazzani AD, Potì E, Genazzani AR. One-year therapy with 10mg/day DHEA alone or in combination with HRT in postmenopausal women: effects on hormonal milieu. Maturitas. 2008 Apr 20;59(4):293-303. https://pubmed.ncbi.nlm.nih.gov/18394829/
4. Panjari M, Davis SR. DHEA therapy for women: effect on sexual function and wellbeing. Hum Reprod Update. 2007 May-Jun;13(3):239-48. https://pubmed.ncbi.nlm.nih.gov/17208951/
5. Genazzani AD, Stomati M, Bernardi F, Pieri M, Rovati L, Genazzani

AR. Long-term low-dose dehydroepiandrosterone oral supplementation in early and late postmenopausal women modulates endocrine parameters and synthesis of neuroactive steroids. Fertil Steril. 2003 Dec;80(6):1495-501. https://pubmed.ncbi.nlm.nih.gov/14667889/

6. Villareal DT, Holloszy JO. Effect of DHEA on abdominal fat and insulin action in elderly women and men: a randomized controlled trial. JAMA. 2004 Nov 10;292(18):2243-8. https://pubmed.ncbi.nlm.nih.gov/15536111/

7. Fathizadeh N, Ebrahimi E, Valiani M, Tavakoli N, Yar MH. Evaluating the effect of magnesium and magnesium plus vitamin B6 supplement on the severity of premenstrual syndrome. Iran J Nurs Midwifery Res. 2010 Dec;15(Suppl 1):401-5. https://www.ncbi.nlm.nih.gov/pmc/articles/PMC3208934/

8. Masoumi SZ, Ataollahi M, Oshvandi K. Effect of Combined Use of Calcium and Vitamin B6 on Premenstrual Syndrome Symptoms: a Randomized Clinical Trial. J Caring Sci. 2016 Mar 1;5(1):67-73. https://www.ncbi.nlm.nih.gov/pmc/articles/PMC4794546/

9. Tully L, Humiston J, Cash A. Oxaloacetate reduces emotional symptoms in premenstrual syndrome (PMS): results of a placebo-controlled, cross-over clinical trial. Obstet Gynecol Sci. 2020 Mar;63(2):195-204. https://pubmed.ncbi.nlm.nih.gov/32206660/

10. Bahrami A, Avan A, Sadeghnia HR, Esmaeili H, Tayefi M, Ghasemi F, Nejati Salehkhani F, Arabpour-Dahoue M, Rastgar-Moghadam A, Ferns GA, Bahrami-Taghanaki H, Ghayour-Mobarhan M. High dose vitamin D supplementation can improve menstrual problems, dysmenorrhea, and premenstrual syndrome in adolescents. Gynecol Endocrinol. 2018 Aug;34(8):659-663. https://pubmed.ncbi.nlm.nih.gov/29447494/

11. Abdi F, Ozgoli G, Rahnemaie FS. A systematic review of the role of vitamin D and calcium in premenstrual syndrome. Obstet Gynecol Sci. 2019 Mar;62(2):73-86. doi: 10.5468/ogs.2019.62.2.73. Epub 2019 Feb 25. Erratum in: Obstet Gynecol Sci. 2020 Mar;63(2):213. https://www.ncbi.nlm.nih.gov/pmc/articles/PMC6422848/

12. Eriksson O, Wall A, Olsson U, Marteinsdottir I, Holstad M, Ågren H, Hartvig P, Långström B, Naessén T. Women with Premenstrual Dysphoria Lack the Seemingly Normal Premenstrual Right-Sided Relative Dominance of 5-HTP-Derived Serotonergic Activity in the Dorsolateral Prefrontal Cortices - A Possible Cause of Disabling Mood Symptoms. PLoS One. 2016 Sep 12;11(9):e0159538. https://www.ncbi.nlm.nih.gov/pmc/articles/PMC5019404/
13. Menkes DB, Coates DC, Fawcett JP. Acute tryptophan depletion aggravates premenstrual syndrome. J Affect Disord. 1994 Sep;32(1):37-44. https://pubmed.ncbi.nlm.nih.gov/7798465/
14. Steinberg S, Annable L, Young SN, Liyanage N. A placebo-controlled clinical trial of L-tryptophan in premenstrual dysphoria. Biol Psychiatry. 1999 Feb 1;45(3):313-20. https://pubmed.ncbi.nlm.nih.gov/10023508/
15. Banderet LE, Lieberman HR. Treatment with tyrosine, a neurotransmitter precursor, reduces environmental stress in humans. Brain Res Bull. 1989 Apr;22(4):759-62. https://pubmed.ncbi.nlm.nih.gov/2736402/
16. Stauffer WR, Lak A, Kobayashi S, Schultz W. Components and characteristics of the dopamine reward utility signal. J Comp Neurol. 2016 Jun 1;524(8):1699-711. https://pubmed.ncbi.nlm.nih.gov/26272220/
17. Portugal-Nunes C, Castanho TC, Amorim L, Moreira PS, Mariz J, Marques F, Sousa N, Santos NC, Palha JA. Iron Status is Associated with Mood, Cognition, and Functional Ability in Older Adults: A Cross-Sectional Study. Nutrients. 2020 Nov 23;12(11):3594. https://pubmed.ncbi.nlm.nih.gov/33238615/
18. Dadkhah H, Ebrahimi E, Fathizadeh N. Evaluating the effects of vitamin D and vitamin E supplement on premenstrual syndrome: A randomized, double-blind, controlled trial. Iran J Nurs Midwifery Res. 2016 Mar-Apr;21(2):159-64.https://www.ncbi.nlm.nih.gov/pmc/articles/PMC4815371/
19. Siahbazi S, Behboudi-Gandevani S, Moghaddam-Banaem L, Montazeri A. Effect of zinc sulfate supplementation on premenstrual

syndrome and health-related quality of life: Clinical randomized controlled trial. J Obstet Gynaecol Res. 2017 May;43(5):887-894. https://pubmed.ncbi.nlm.nih.gov/28188965/
20. Sohrabi N, Kashanian M, Ghafoori SS, Malakouti SK. Evaluation of the effect of omega-3 fatty acids in the treatment of premenstrual syndrome: "a pilot trial". Complement Ther Med. 2013 Jun;21(3):141-6. https://pubmed.ncbi.nlm.nih.gov/23642943/
21. Mohammadi MM, Dehghan Nayeri N, Mashhadi M, Varaei S. Effect of omega-3 fatty acids on premenstrual syndrome: A systematic review and meta-analysis. J Obstet Gynaecol Res. 2022 Jun;48(6):1293-1305. https://pubmed.ncbi.nlm.nih.gov/35266254/
22. Gioffrè, W., Ditto, A., Tripodi, A., & Ciatto, S. (1998). Danazol versus Cabergolina for the treatment of Cyclic mastalgia. European Journal of Cancer, 34. https://pjs.com.pk/journal_pdfs/jan_mar07/03.pdf
23. Hijová E, Kuzma J, Strojný L, Bomba A, Bertková I, Chmelárová A, Hertelyová Z, Benetinová V, Štofilová J, Ambro Ľ. Ability of Lactobacillus plantarum LS/07 to modify intestinal enzymes activity in chronic diseases prevention. Acta Biochim Pol. 2017;64(1):113-116. https://pubmed.ncbi.nlm.nih.gov/27824363/
24. Ma T, Jin H, Kwok LY, Sun Z, Liong MT, Zhang H. Probiotic consumption relieved human stress and anxiety symptoms possibly via modulating the neuroactive potential of the gut microbiota. Neurobiol Stress. 2021 Jan 12;14:100294. https://pubmed.ncbi.nlm.nih.gov/33511258/
25. Tully L, Humiston J, Cash A. Oxaloacetate reduces emotional symptoms in premenstrual syndrome (PMS): results of a placebo-controlled, cross-over clinical trial. Obstet Gynecol Sci. 2020 Mar;63(2):195-204. https://pubmed.ncbi.nlm.nih.gov/32206660/
26. Schmidt K, Weber N, Steiner M, Meyer N, Dubberke A, Rutenberg D, Hellhammer J. A lecithin phosphatidylserine and phosphatidic acid complex (PAS) reduces symptoms of the premenstrual syndrome (PMS): Results of a randomized, placebo-controlled, double-blind clinical trial. Clin Nutr ESPEN. 2018 Apr;24:22-30. https://pubm

ed.ncbi.nlm.nih.gov/29576358/
27. Rajabi F, Rahimi M, Sharbafchizadeh MR, Tarrahi MJ. Saffron for the Management of Premenstrual Dysphoric Disorder: A Randomized Controlled Trial. Adv Biomed Res. 2020 Oct 30;9:60. https://www.ncbi.nlm.nih.gov/pmc/articles/PMC7792881/
28. Zamani M, Neghab N, Torabian S. Therapeutic effect of Vitex agnus castus in patients with premenstrual syndrome. Acta Med Iran. 2012;50(2):101-6. https://pubmed.ncbi.nlm.nih.gov/22359078/
29. Verkaik S, Kamperman AM, van Westrhenen R, Schulte PFJ. The treatment of premenstrual syndrome with preparations of Vitex agnus castus: a systematic review and meta-analysis. Am J Obstet Gynecol. 2017 Aug;217(2):150-166. https://pubmed.ncbi.nlm.nih.gov/28237870/
30. Csupor D, Lantos T, Hegyi P, Benkő R, Viola R, Gyöngyi Z, Csécsei P, Tóth B, Vasas A, Márta K, Rostás I, Szentesi A, Matuz M. Vitex agnus-castus in premenstrual syndrome: A meta-analysis of double-blind randomised controlled trials. Complement Ther Med. 2019 Dec;47:102190. https://pubmed.ncbi.nlm.nih.gov/31780016/
31. Khayat S, Fanaei H, Kheirkhah M, Moghadam ZB, Kasaeian A, Javadimehr M. Curcumin attenuates severity of premenstrual syndrome symptoms: A randomized, double-blind, placebo-controlled trial. Complement Ther Med. 2015 Jun;23(3):318-24. https://pubmed.ncbi.nlm.nih.gov/26051565/
32. Khayat S, Kheirkhah M, Behboodi Moghadam Z, Fanaei H, Kasaeian A, Javadimehr M. Effect of treatment with ginger on the severity of premenstrual syndrome symptoms. ISRN Obstet Gynecol. 2014 May 4;2014:792708. https://pubmed.ncbi.nlm.nih.gov/24944825/
33. Ozgoli G, Selselei EA, Mojab F, Majd HA. A randomized, placebo-controlled trial of Ginkgo biloba L. in treatment of premenstrual syndrome. J Altern Complement Med. 2009 Aug;15(8):845-51. https://pubmed.ncbi.nlm.nih.gov/19678774/
34. Tamborini A, Taurelle R. Intérêt de l'extrait standardisé de Ginkgo biloba (EGb 761) dans la prise en charge des symptômes congestifs du

syndrome prémenstruel [Value of standardized Ginkgo biloba extract (EGb 761) in the management of congestive symptoms of premenstrual syndrome]. Rev Fr Gynecol Obstet. 1993 Jul-Sep;88(7-9):447-57. French. https://pubmed.ncbi.nlm.nih.gov/8235261/

35. Chaurasiya ND, Zhao J, Pandey P, Doerksen RJ, Muhammad I, Tekwani BL. Selective Inhibition of Human Monoamine Oxidase B by Acacetin 7-Methyl Ether Isolated from Turnera diffusa (Damiana). Molecules. 2019 Feb 23;24(4):810. https://pubmed.ncbi.nlm.nih.gov/30813423/

36. Edgar Romualdo EG, Lilia AM, Rafael SG, Alfredo SM. Antioxidant effects of damiana (Turnera diffusa Willd. ex Schult.) in kidney mitochondria from streptozotocin-diabetic rats. Nat Prod Res. 2018 Dec;32(23):2840-2843.https://pubmed.ncbi.nlm.nih.gov/28948849/

37. Crippa JA, Guimarães FS, Campos AC, Zuardi AW. Translational Investigation of the Therapeutic Potential of Cannabidiol (CBD): Toward a New Age. Front Immunol. 2018 Sep 21;9:2009. https://www.ncbi.nlm.nih.gov/pmc/articles/PMC6161644/

38. Khalesi ZB, Beiranvand SP, Bokaie M. Efficacy of Chamomile in the Treatment of Premenstrual Syndrome: A Systematic Review. J Pharmacopuncture. 2019 Dec;22(4):204-209. https://pubmed.ncbi.nlm.nih.gov/31970017/

39. Matsumoto T, Asakura H, Hayashi T. Does lavender aromatherapy alleviate premenstrual emotional symptoms?: a randomized crossover trial. Biopsychosoc Med. 2013 May 31;7:12. https://www.ncbi.nlm.nih.gov/pmc/articles/PMC3674979/

40. Donelli D, Antonelli M, Bellinazzi C, Gensini GF, Firenzuoli F. Effects of lavender on anxiety: A systematic review and meta-analysis. Phytomedicine. 2019 Dec;65:153099. https://pubmed.ncbi.nlm.nih.gov/31655395/

41. Portincasa P, Bonfrate L, de Bari O, Lembo A, Ballou S. Irritable bowel syndrome and diet. Gastroenterol Rep (Oxf). 2017 Feb;5(1):11-19. https://www.ncbi.nlm.nih.gov/pmc/articles/PMC5444258/

42. Ostad SN, Soodi M, Shariffzadeh M, Khorshidi N, Marzban H. The effect of fennel essential oil on uterine contraction as a model for

dysmenorrhea, pharmacology and toxicology study. J Ethnopharmacol. 2001 Aug;76(3):299-304.https://pubmed.ncbi.nlm.nih.gov/11448553/

43. Portincasa P, Bonfrate L, de Bari O, Lembo A, Ballou S. Irritable bowel syndrome and diet. Gastroenterol Rep (Oxf). 2017 Feb;5(1):11-19. https://www.ncbi.nlm.nih.gov/pmc/articles/PMC5444258/
44. Sildenafil. National Library of Medicine. https://pubmed.ncbi.nlm.nih.gov/?term=sildenafil
45. Perimenopause. National Library of Medicine. https://pubmed.ncbi.nlm.nih.gov/?term=perimenopause
46. Burger H, Woods NF, Dennerstein L, Alexander JL, Kotz K, Richardson G. Nomenclature and endocrinology of menopause and perimenopause. Expert Rev Neurother. 2007 Nov;7(11 Suppl):S35-43. https://pubmed.ncbi.nlm.nih.gov/18039067/
47. Dahlgren MK, El-Abboud C, Lambros AM, Sagar KA, Smith RT, Gruber SA. A survey of medical cannabis use during perimenopause and postmenopause. Menopause. 2022 Sep 1;29(9):1028-1036. https://pubmed.ncbi.nlm.nih.gov/35917529/
48. Prior JC, Hitchcock CL, Shirin S, Hale G, Goshtasebi A. Don't ignore perimenopause. CMAJ. 2023 Jul 31;195(29):E987. https://www.ncbi.nlm.nih.gov/pmc/articles/PMC10395791/
49. Sussman M, Trocio J, Best C, Mirkin S, Bushmakin AG, Yood R, Friedman M, Menzin J, Louie M. Prevalence of menopausal symptoms among mid-life women: findings from electronic medical records. BMC Womens Health. 2015 Aug 13;15:58. https://www.ncbi.nlm.nih.gov/pmc/articles/PMC4542113/
50. Ayers B, Hunter MS. Health-related quality of life of women with menopausal hot flushes and night sweats. Climacteric. 2013 Apr;16(2):235-9. https://pubmed.ncbi.nlm.nih.gov/22809134/
51. MailOnline, A. H. for. (2015, June 9). Menopause symptoms depend on where a woman lives: Those in the UK, US and Canada suffer the most - particularly in the bedroom - and Italians and Sweden the least. Daily Mail Online. https://www.dailymail.co.uk/health/article-3116972/

Symptoms-menopause-depend-woman-LIVES-UK-Canada-suffer-particularly-bedroom-Italians-Sweden-least.html

52. Complementary and alternative medicine: Myths and truths: Pharmaceutical society of singapore. Complementary and Alternative Medicine: Myths and Truths | Pharmaceutical Society of Singapore. https://www.pss.org.sg/know-your-medicines/safe-use-medicines/complementary-and-alternative-medicine-myths-and-truths

53. Kalhan M, Singhania K, Choudhary P, Verma S, Kaushal P, Singh T. Prevalence of Menopausal Symptoms and its Effect on Quality of Life among Rural Middle Aged Women (40-60 Years) of Haryana, India. Int J Appl Basic Med Res. 2020 Jul-Sep;10(3):183-188. https://www.ncbi.nlm.nih.gov/pmc/articles/PMC7534715/

54. Harvey Chim, Bee Huat Iain Tan, Chia Chun Ang, Ee Ming Darryl Chew, Yap Seng Chong, Seang Mei Saw. The prevalence of menopausal symptoms in a community in Singapore. Maturitas. 2002. 41(4); 275-282. https://www.sciencedirect.com/science/article/abs/pii/S0378512201002997

55. Thurston RC, El Khoudary SR, Sutton-Tyrrell K, Crandall CJ, Sternfeld B, Joffe H, Gold EB, Selzer F, Matthews KA. Vasomotor symptoms and insulin resistance in the study of women's health across the nation. J Clin Endocrinol Metab. 2012 Oct;97(10):3487-94. https://pubmed.ncbi.nlm.nih.gov/22851488/

56. Sauer T, Tottenham LS, Ethier A, Gordon JL. Perimenopausal vasomotor symptoms and the cortisol awakening response. Menopause. 2020 Nov;27(11):1322-1327. https://pubmed.ncbi.nlm.nih.gov/33110049/

57. Gordon JL, Rubinow DR, Thurston RC, Paulson J, Schmidt PJ, Girdler SS. Cardiovascular, hemodynamic, neuroendocrine, and inflammatory markers in women with and without vasomotor symptoms. Menopause. 2016 Nov;23(11):1189-1198. https://www.ncbi.nlm.nih.gov/pmc/articles/PMC5079797/

58. Carpenter JS, Tisdale JE, Larson JC, Sheng Y, Chen CX, Von Ah D, Kovacs R, Reed SD, Thurston RC, Guthrie KA. MsFLASH analysis of

diurnal salivary cortisol and palpitations in peri- and postmenopausal women. Menopause. 2021 Nov 29;29(2):144-150. https://pubmed.ncbi.nlm.nih.gov/35084374/

59. Shahnazi M, Nahaee J, Mohammad-Alizadeh-Charandabi S, Bayati-payan S. Effect of black cohosh (cimicifuga racemosa) on vasomotor symptoms in postmenopausal women: a randomized clinical trial. J Caring Sci. 2013 Jun 1;2(2):105-13. https://www.ncbi.nlm.nih.gov/pmc/articles/PMC4161092/\

60. Albertazzi P. Noradrenergic and serotonergic modulation to treat vasomotor symptoms. J Br Menopause Soc. 2006 Mar;12(1):7-11. https://pubmed.ncbi.nlm.nih.gov/16513016/

61. Nahidi F, Zare E, Mojab F, Alavi-Majd H. Effects of licorice on relief and recurrence of menopausal hot flashes. Iran J Pharm Res. 2012 Spring;11(2):541-8. PMID: 24250477; PMCID: PMC3832176. https://www.ncbi.nlm.nih.gov/pmc/articles/PMC3832176/

62. Ataei-Almanghadim K, Farshbaf-Khalili A, Ostadrahimi AR, Shaseb E, Mirghafourvand M. The effect of oral capsule of curcumin and vitamin E on the hot flashes and anxiety in postmenopausal women: A triple blind randomised controlled trial. Complement Ther Med. 2020 Jan;48:102267. https://pubmed.ncbi.nlm.nih.gov/31987231/

63. Ibrahim RM, Hamdan NS, Ismail M, Saini SM, Abd Rashid SN, Abd Latiff L, Mahmud R. Protective Effects of Nigella sativa on Metabolic Syndrome in Menopausal Women. Adv Pharm Bull. 2014;4(1):29-33. https://www.ncbi.nlm.nih.gov/pmc/articles/PMC3885365/

64. An edible for hot flashes? some women use cannabis to manage menopause. (n.d.-a). https://www.washingtonpost.com/wellness/2022/10/21/cannabis-menopause-symptoms

65. Mauskop A, Varughese J. Why all migraine patients should be treated with magnesium. J Neural Transm (Vienna). 2012 May;119(5):575-9. https://pubmed.ncbi.nlm.nih.gov/22426836/

66. Charleston L 4th, Khalil S, Young WB. Carnitine Responsive Migraine Headache Syndrome: Case Report and Review of the Literature. Curr Pain Headache Rep. 2021 Mar 23;25(4):26. https://pubmed.ncbi.nlm.

nih.gov/33755806/

67. Namazi N, Heshmati J, Tarighat-Esfanjani A. Supplementation with Riboflavin (Vitamin B2) for Migraine Prophylaxis in Adults and Children: A Review. Int J Vitam Nutr Res. 2015;85(1-2):79-87. https://pubmed.ncbi.nlm.nih.gov/26780280/

68. Sadeghi O, Nasiri M, Maghsoudi Z, Pahlavani N, Rezaie M, Askari G. Effects of pyridoxine supplementation on severity, frequency and duration of migraine attacks in migraine patients with aura: A double-blind randomized clinical trial study in Iran. Iran J Neurol. 2015 Apr 4;14(2):74-80. https://www.ncbi.nlm.nih.gov/pmc/articles/PMC4449397/

69. Shoeibi A, Olfati N, Soltani Sabi M, Salehi M, Mali S, Akbari Oryani M. Effectiveness of coenzyme Q10 in prophylactic treatment of migraine headache: an open-label, add-on, controlled trial. Acta Neurol Belg. 2017 Mar;117(1):103-109. https://pubmed.ncbi.nlm.nih.gov/27670440/

70. Lipton RB, Göbel H, Einhäupl KM, Wilks K, Mauskop A. Petasites hybridus root (butterbur) is an effective preventive treatment for migraine. Neurology. 2004 Dec 28;63(12):2240-4. https://pubmed.ncbi.nlm.nih.gov/15623680/

71. Ernst E, Pittler MH. The efficacy and safety of feverfew (Tanacetum parthenium L.): an update of a systematic review. Public Health Nutr. 2000 Dec;3(4A):509-14. https://pubmed.ncbi.nlm.nih.gov/11276299/

72. Nappi RE, Merki-Feld GS, Terreno E, Pellegrinelli A, Viana M. Hormonal contraception in women with migraine: is progestogen-only contraception a better choice? J Headache Pain. 2013 Aug 1;14(1):66. https://www.ncbi.nlm.nih.gov/pmc/articles/PMC3735427/

73. Peikert A, et al. Prophylaxis of migraine with oral magnesium: results from a prospective, multi-center, placebo-controlled and double-blind randomized study. Cephalalgia. 1996;16(257-63).https://pubmed.ncbi.nlm.nih.gov/8902254/

74. Chayasirisobhon S. Use of a pine bark extract and antioxidant vitamin

combination product as therapy for migraine in patients refractory to pharmacologic medication. Headache. 2006 May;46(5):788-93. https://pubmed.ncbi.nlm.nih.gov/16643582/

75. Rafieian-Kopaei M, Hasanpour-Dehkordi A, Lorigooini Z, Deris F, Solati K, Mahdiyeh F. Comparing the Effect of Intranasal Lidocaine 4% with Peppermint Essential Oil Drop 1.5% on Migraine Attacks: A Double-Blind Clinical Trial. Int J Prev Med. 2019 Jul 5;10:121. https://www.ncbi.nlm.nih.gov/pmc/articles/PMC6647908/

Eight

Chapter 8

Diet for A Healthy Period

A cornerstone to having a healthy period must include healthy meals that nourish the uterus as reviewed in Chapter 9. That is why I'm giving you a template for meals that you can easily include but also foods that you should try to limit and avoid.

In this chapter, I will also give you a 2-week meal plan and recipes for your meal plan, as well as other tips to maintain your healthiest hormonal self.

Foods to Avoid or Limit

Simply put, if a food or drink comes in plastic or a shiny package or can, you need to highly consider avoiding it. Not only is the plastic packaging disruptive to hormones, the odds are, they add in a lot of preservatives and refine these foods so much that they hardly count as food.

Typically the things to leave on the grocery store shelf are cookies, cakes, pies, candies, chips, crackers, sodas, energy drinks, breads, packaged meals, most pastas, and pre-prepared side dishes, even in the deli.

Or just avoid the center aisles of the store, with the exception of tinned meats, canned vegetables, and the occasional condiment that might be ok to include.

The Meal Balance

For optimal hormonal health, you should strive for around 30-50% of your calories from natural fat. This would mean that your protein intake should be at 25-35% with carbohydrates ranging from 15-40% of your calories. These carbs need to be from real food sources, not snacks!

Your plate is going to be filled with following: at least half of the plate with olive oil and other healthy fats, eggs or grass fed meats, fish, and the like to give plenty of healthy fats and proteins, with vegetables filling up most of the rest of the plate. Round it out with a little probiotic-rich cheese or plain whole-milk yogurt. When needed, add in some gut-friendly carbs like fruit, sweet potatoes, other root veggies, or fermented rice. This shouldn't be more than a quarter of your plate. Then, if you get munchies later, grab some walnuts, almonds, or macadamia nuts. Another good option for a balanced dish is curries or a stew.

Don't worry too much; I will get into some recipes that make my life, and hopefully help make your life, easier to get the balance right.

2-Week Meal Plan

I'm not going to lie; I'm not much of a planner, especially when it comes to a week full of menus. This is because my life is a bit different every day with a bunch of moving parts. For this reason, I tend to keep staples on hand that I know are healthy and that I know that I like to eat. But some people function best with a plan and a list, so the next sections are for you to get some ideas of how you might structure your week.

Some of these meals may be an adventure of new foods but I encourage you to try some of them-especially the ones that contain liver in them. The taste of these is going to surprise you in a pleasant way, at least I hope!

Keep in mind that flexibility can be built into these meal plans. For example, I give some suggestions of teas for you that help promote a healthy period. Don't worry if you don't like tea; you can supplement these herbs instead if you wish. But you might be surprised that if you make iced tea out of these herbal infusions you might like the taste of all of them. And teas are simply infusions that contain very small amounts of active herbs, so they aren't going to give you too much of any single ingredient. They probably aren't enough to change your periods alone unless you have them consistently at each meal. As a bonus tea will help improve hydration.

Last but not least, if you know you don't tolerate some of these foods, simply don't eat them. We are all different and as such, I can't pretend that all foods are going to work for you. However, if you have been eliminating the major gut offenders like gluten, you may be surprised that you can tolerate foods that you previously thought you couldn't. For example, after I eliminated gluten from my diet for a month, I realized that raw broccoli was totally fine in my diet where it previously wasn't. This is because the gluten was damaging my gut, and as such, foods like raw broccoli bugged me. Once I healed my gut, broccoli is not only well-tolerated, it feels great when I eat it. Food isn't a straight line, in other words, it's a journey and an experience that can change depending on a lot of things you do or don't do.

If the food listed in the meal plan has an asterisk * by it, this means there is a recipe included for it in the recipe section. And above all, please don't get caught up too heavily in stressing over doing this exactly like I suggest. These are only ideas to help you understand that meals can and should be tasty, nutritious, and easy to make.

This plan includes two meals a day, but if you need a third meal, you can simply eat leftovers. To accomplish this, consider making double portions of these dishes in the recipe section.

Week 1

Sunday
  Meal 1

- *Berry Yogurt "Dessert"
- *Green salad with Lemony Dressing
- Can of sardines or yellowfin tuna with olive oil
- Tulsi tea

Meal 2

- *Meatballs with Nourishing Beef Liver
- *Fermented rice
- Fresh orange wedges
- Mixed Nuts
- Chamomile tea

Monday

Meal 1

- *Leftover meatballs and fermented rice
- *Salad with super greens/Lemony Dressing
- Fresh berries
- Raspberry leaf tea

Meal 2

- *Creamy chicken with mushrooms
- *Sweet potatoes, air fryer style
- *Fermented veggies
- Licorice root tea

Tuesday

Meal 1

- *Broccoli salad
- *Leftover chicken with mushrooms
- Leftover sweet potatoes air fryer
- Herbal tea

Meal 2

- *Burger bowls
- *Leftover broccoli salad
- Nuts
- Tulsi tea

Wednesday

Meal 1

- *Salsa poached eggs

- *Fermented veggies
- 1/2 avocado
- *Skillet potatoes
- Red raspberry leaf tea

Meal 2

- *Salmon bowl
- *Sweet potato hash
- Chamomile tea

Thursday
Meal 1

- *Leftover salmon bowl
- *Sauerkraut
- Green salad
- *Leftover hash
- Tulsi tea

Meal 2

- *Butter chicken
- Potatoes of choice
- *Buttery Sauteed Beets
- Red raspberry leaf tea

Friday
Meal 1

- *Leftover butter chicken, potatoes, and beets
- Mixed nuts
- Fresh apple

- Herbal tea of choice

Meal 2

- *Fluffy Egg Muffins
- 1/2 avocado
- *Arugula with Lemony Dressing
- *Leftover potatoes/cheese
- Tulsi tea

Saturday
Meal 1

- *Tuna salad on greens
- Plantain chips
- *Fermented vegetables
- Red raspberry leaf tea

Meal 2

- *Honey-Garlic Shrimp and Broccoli
- *Sauerkraut
- Fresh berries
- Chamomile tea

Week 2

Sunday
Meal 1

- *Leftover Garlic Shrimp and Broccoli
- *Sauerkraut
- Damiana tea

Meal 2

- *Sheet pan sausage and veggies
- Baked Brie
- Pomegranate or berries
- Chamomile tea

Monday
Meal 1

- *Leftover egg muffins
- Fresh or frozen berries
- Red raspberry leaf tea

Meal 2

- *Pepper steak in the slow cooker
- 1/2 avocado
- Fresh fruit
- Chamomile tea

Tuesday
Meal 1

- *Leftover pepper steak
- Leftover baked Brie
- Tulsi tea

Meal 2

- *Chicken Vegetable Soup
- Mixed nuts
- Sage tea

Wednesday

Meal 1

- *Versatile Egg Pie
- Fresh berries and whole milk yogurt
- Peppermint tea

Meal 2

- *Healthy chicken nuggets
- *Green salad with lemony dressing
- Baked sweet potato with cultured sour cream
- Red raspberry leaf tea

Thursday

Meal 1

- Leftover chicken nuggets
- Leftover sweet potato
- Avocado half
- Ginger tea

Meal 2

- *Liver, Vodka, and Onions
- *Roasted vegetables with Parmesan
- Red raspberry leaf tea

Friday
  Meal 1

- *Leftover chicken vegetable soup
- *Sauteed potatoes
- Green tea

Meal 2

- *Greek salad with Chicken/Gyro Meat
- Fresh orange slices
- Chamomile tea

Saturday
  Meal 1

- *Leftover Greek salad
- Mixed nuts
- Ginger tea

Meal 2

- *Salmon with pesto
- *Fermented rice
- *Sauteed broccoli
- Red raspberry leaf tea

Nine

Chapter 9

Recipes

This chapter contains 32 recipes that can help you heal on your journey to healthier periods. From my kitchen to yours, I hope you enjoy these dishes!

Section 1: Egg Dishes and Brunch Dishes

Chapter 9

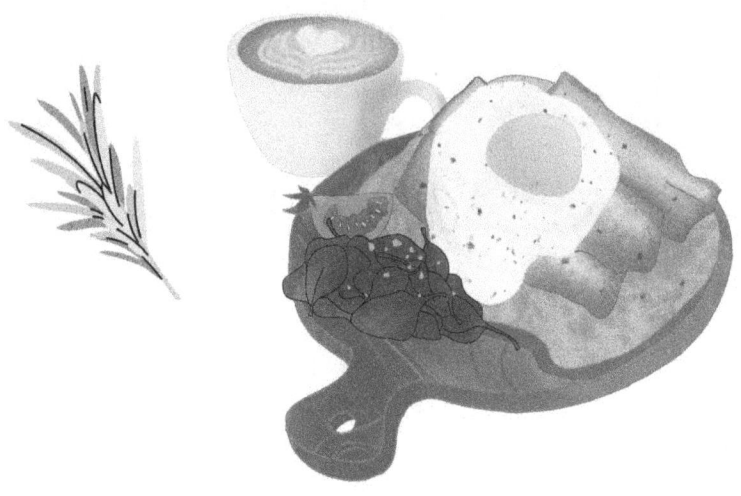

Here are 3 simple and delicious egg dishes that I love. When you cook eggs, you can be as creative as you want to be. Personally, I love keeping it simple for brunch by making a simple egg scramble with fresh sauerkraut, some sour cream, and some salsa on top. Don't knock it until you try it! The savory combination is amazing.

Fluffy Egg Muffins

Total time: 30 minutes Serves: 3-4

Eggs make for the easiest meals and happen to be very hormone-healthy. This dish is tasty served with some salsa and a side of some fresh fruit like fresh berries. Fruit complements eggs well in terms of digestion because of their natural enzyme content. It also goes well with Sauteed Potatoes on page 242. I recommend that you use a ceramic muffin pan to avoid hormonal-disrupting coatings or suspect metals used in many muffin tins.

- 8 large pasture-raised eggs
- 1/2 cup whole milk organic cottage cheese
- 1/4 tsp Himalayan salt
- 1/4 tsp pepper
- 1.5 cups chopped or shredded add-ins, (I like tomatoes, sliced olives, chopped bell peppers, onions, mushrooms, cheese, or spinach)
- Extra virgin olive oil
- Ceramic muffin pan

1. Preheat the oven to 375°F (190°C). Liberally grease the tins with olive oil.
2. Place 2 tbsp of add-ins into each muffin tin.
3. Add the eggs, cottage cheese, salt, and pepper to a large blender. Purée for about 30 seconds or until smooth.
4. Pour the egg mixture into the wells of the muffin tin, dividing evenly between each well. It should fill them almost to the top.
5. Bake for 18 minutes, or just until the centers no longer look wet, and they are barely golden around the edges. Avoid overcooking, as they'll become spongy.
6. Allow the muffins to cool in the tin just enough to handle, then loosen them gently with a knife and remove them from the tin. Allow them to finish cooling on a wire rack.

Chapter 9

Versatile Egg Pie Recipe

Total Time: 30 minutes Serves 3 to 4

This isn't a pie at all, but an easy oven-baked egg dish that is super quick to make. Growing up, we had frittata all the time, but we called it egg pie. I like both names, but the name egg pie makes me reminisce about home. Here is a basic egg pie recipe plus 3 variations that you will love. You can also add in meat of your choice if you wish.

Basic Frittata Recipe:

- 6 large pasture-raised eggs, use 8 eggs for a 12-inch skillet
- ¼ cup whole milk
- 2 garlic cloves, minced
- ¼ tsp Himalayan salt, more for sprinkling
- Freshly ground black pepper
- Extra-virgin olive oil, for the pan
- Choose ingredients for one of the variations below:

Broccoli version: add in chopped green onions, about 2 cups chopped broccoli, and ¼ cup feta.

Asparagus version: add in about ½ cup chopped green onions, ½ cup chopped asparagus, ½ cup peas, ½ cup mini mozzarella balls, ½ cup Parmesan.

Mushroom version: ½ cup chopped green onions, 8-12 ounces chopped mushrooms of your choice, ¼ cup tarragon, ½ cup Parmesan cheese.

1. Preheat the oven to 400°F.
2. Whisk the eggs, milk, garlic, and salt until well combined. Set aside. Follow the instructions to make one of the vegetable variations below:

3. **Broccoli:** Heat 1 tablespoon olive oil in a cast-iron skillet over medium heat. Add the onions, broccoli, and a pinch of salt and pepper and cook, stirring occasionally, until the broccoli is tender but still bright green, about 5 to 8 minutes. Add the eggs and sprinkle with the feta; bake for 15 to 20 minutes or until the eggs are set. Season to taste and serve.
4. **Asparagus:** Heat ½ tablespoon olive oil in a cast-iron skillet over medium heat. Add the scallions, asparagus, and a pinch of salt and pepper and cook, stirring occasionally, until the asparagus is tender but still bright green, about 5 minutes. Add the peas, then add the egg mixture and gently shake the pan to distribute. Add the mozzarella and Parmesan and bake for 15 to 20 minutes or until the eggs are set. Season to taste and serve.
5. **Mushroom**: Heat 1 tablespoon olive oil in a cast-iron skillet over medium heat. Add the shallot, and a pinch of salt and pepper and cook until beginning to soften, about 3 minutes. Add the mushrooms, stir, and cook until soft and tender, about 8 minutes, stirring only occasionally. Stir in the tarragon, then add the egg mixture and gently shake the pan to distribute. Sprinkle with Parmesan and bake for 15 to 20 minutes or until the eggs are set. Season to taste and serve.

Salsa Poached Eggs

Eggs are healthy with lots of hormone-supporting nutrients, but the taste for me can be boring. This adaptation of eggs spices it up a bit for a tasty and nutritious light meal. Full of antioxidant-rich spices and herbs to support hormonal health.

Total time: 25 minutes Serves 1-2

- 1/2 white onion, minced
- 2 cloves garlic, minced
- 2 Tbsp olive oil

- 1-15 oz. can fire-roasted diced tomatoes
- 1-4 oz. can diced green chilies
- 2 Tbsp tomato paste
- 1/2 tsp cumin, freshly ground if possible
- ½ tsp coriander, freshly ground if possible
- 1/8 tsp cayenne
- 1/2 tsp Himalayan salt
- 1/4 tsp freshly cracked black pepper
- 1/2 cup water
- 4 large pasture-raised eggs
- 2 green onions, sliced
- 2 Tbsp chopped cilantro

1. Add the onions and garlic to a deep skillet with the olive oil and saute over medium heat until the onions are soft, about 5 minutes.
2. Mix in the diced tomatoes with juices, green chilies with juices, tomato paste, cumin, coriander, cayenne, salt, pepper, and water. Stir to combine.
3. Allow the salsa to come up to a simmer, stirring occasionally and simmer for about 10 minutes until it is slightly thickened.
4. Use the back of a spoon to make four indentations in the sauce. Crack one egg into each indentation.
5. Place a lid on the skillet, turn the heat down to medium-low, and let the eggs simmer in the sauce for 7-10 minutes, or until they reach your desired doneness.
6. Once the eggs are cooked, garnish with sliced green onion and chopped cilantro, then serve with your side of choice such as avocado or some hash browns. To keep it low carb, you can simply serve it with an avocado.

Section 2: Salads and Sides

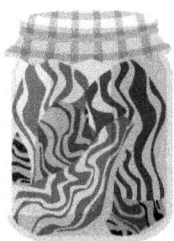
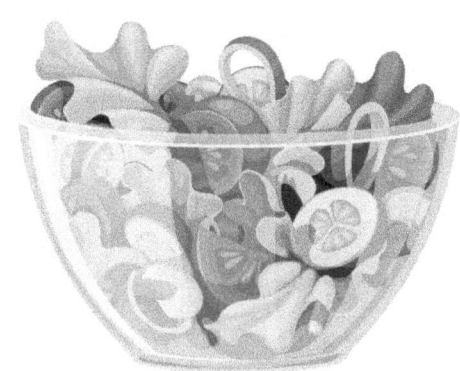

Here are 12 side dishes and salad recipes that help provide antioxidant-rich foods that are helpful for most anyone on their journey to better health.

Lemony Dressing

The best salad dressings are often the simplest. You can make many variations of this dressing and serve it on just about anything you can imagine, such as pan-seared chicken, fish, steaks, as well as many types of salads.

Total time: 5 minutes Serves 1-2

- 3 tbsp extra-virgin olive oil
- Juice of half of a lemon
- Pinch of salt and pepper

Optional but encouraged ingredients:

- 1 tsp Dijon mustard
- 1 tbsp freshly chopped tarragon or basil

Combine the above ingredients. You can triple the recipe and keep it in the refrigerator for up to a week.

Tuna Salad on Greens

The quickest meals can be the healthiest as is the case for this salad. I make a version of this about every week and sometimes I substitute salad shrimp for tuna. The cilantro helps gently remove heavy metals from the body which in turn helps normalize hormonal levels.

Serves 1 Total time: 5 minutes

- 5-6 large lettuce leaves such as butter lettuce or Romaine lettuce
- 1 can yellowfin tuna or light tuna
- 1 avocado, cubed
- 5-6 radishes, thinly sliced
- ½ red bell pepper, cubed
- 2 celery stalks, sliced
- 2 mini cucumbers, sliced
- 1/4 white onion, chopped
- 1/2 cup fresh cilantro or parsley, chopped

Salad Dressing:

- 2 tbsp extra virgin olive oil
- 1 tsp apple cider vinegar with the mother
- 3 cloves garlic, minced
- 1 tbsp chopped cilantro or parsley
- Himalayan salt and freshly grounded pepper, to taste
- pinch red pepper flakes (optional)

Toss all the vegetables together on a plate. Top with the crumbled tuna. In a small bowl whisk the salad dressing ingredients. Pour dressing over the tuna salad and give it a little mix. Season to taste and add more fresh herbs like cilantro or dill.

Greek Salad

This salad is versatile and to make it a complete meal, toss in some gyro meat or sauteed chicken.

Total Time: 15 minutes Serves 4

Dressing

- ¼ cup extra-virgin olive oil
- 3 tbsp red wine vinegar
- 1 garlic clove, minced
- 1 tsp dried oregano, more for sprinkling
- ½ tsp Dijon mustard
- ¼ tsp sea salt
- Freshly ground black pepper

For the salad

- 1 cucumber, cut lengthwise, peeled, seeded, and sliced about ¼-inch thick
- 2 cups halved cherry tomatoes or other types of tomatoes cut up if you wish
- 5 ounces feta cheese, cut into ½ inch pieces
- ⅓ cup thinly sliced red onion
- ¼ cup pitted Kalamata olives
- ⅓ cup fresh mint leaves (optional)

1. Dressing: whisk together the olive oil, vinegar, garlic, oregano, mustard, salt, and several grinds of pepper.
2. On a large platter, arrange the cucumber, tomatoes, feta cheese, red onions, and olives. Drizzle with the dressing and very gently toss. Sprinkle a few generous pinches of oregano and top with the mint leaves if you wish.

Broccoli Salad

Broccoli salad is an underrated side because it has lots of hormone-balancing compounds in it and it tastes so delicious. This recipe combines sweet, sour, salt, and bitter flavors which should please almost everyone!

Serves: 3-5 Total time: 10 minutes

5-6 cups broccoli florets

- 1 cup sharp cheddar cheese shredded
- ¼ cup raisins or dried cherries

- ½ cup cooked and crumbled uncured bacon
- ½ cup salted sunflower seeds
- ⅓ cup red or white onion diced into small pieces

Dressing

- 3 tbsp extra virgin olive oil
- 2 tbsp apple cider vinegar with the mother
- 2 tbsp real maple syrup
- 1 tbsp Dijon mustard
- ¼ tsp Himalayan salt
- ½ tsp black pepper

Instructions

1. Combine broccoli florets, cheddar cheese, dried fruit, bacon, sunflower seeds, and onion in a large bowl.
2. In a separate, small bowl, whisk together the dressing ingredients.
3. Pour dressing over broccoli combination and toss or stir well.
4. Broccoli salad may be served immediately, but for the best flavor refrigerate for at least one hour before serving. Make sure to toss broccoli salad thoroughly again before serving.
5. Keep refrigerated if not consumed right away.

Buttery Sauteed Beets

If you are like me, butter and beets together are a marriage of joy for my taste buds. Beets are great for gut health and can boost energy by supporting nitric oxide levels in the body. They also dampen inflammation which helps hormone balance.

- 1 ½ pounds of beets, diced into ½ inch cubes
- 4 tbsp butter
- 1 onion, chopped
- Fresh herbs

Melt the butter in a saucepan. Saute beets and onions over medium heat until desired softness, about 8-12 minutes. Top with fresh herbs of your choice. Note: you can use this recipe for sweet potatoes instead of beets if you prefer.

Sauerkraut Recipe

This recipe was originally posted on my website here: https://thehealthyrd.com/22-raw-sauerkraut-benefits-that-may-change-your-life/ I encourage you to check out my post because it talks about the countless benefits of fermenting foods and sauerkraut in particular.

What you need:

- 1 head of red cabbage or green cabbage, preferably organic
- non-iodized salt, about 1 tbsp
- wide-mouth quart-size mason jar
- vegetable pounder*

1. Peel off the outer leaves of a cabbage, then slice the cabbage finely with a sharp knife on a cutting board. *I prefer to use a slicing food

processor to slice the cabbage because I don't risk cutting my fingers!
2. Then, massage the chopped cabbage with salt, wait 45 minutes, and massage the cabbage again. You can use a vegetable pounder for this task as well.
3. Next, tamp down the salted cabbage with a vegetable pounder in a large quart-size wide-mouth mason jar to release the cabbage juice. Make sure the liquid or brine covers all the cabbage at this point.
4. Place a cabbage leaf cut to the size of the jar on top of the cabbage to help keep the sliced cabbage submerged.
5. Place a small glass weight on top to weigh it all down, such as a very small glass jar. Or you can use a whole cabbage leaf on the top of the sauerkraut to keep the vegetables submerged in the brine. This step is essential so don't skip it otherwise you may end up with moldy sauerkraut.
6. Loosely place a lid on top, making sure it is loose enough so gasses can be released from the jar.
7. Store the brined cabbage in low light and at room temperature for 7-14 days, and make sure to check on it every day to make sure all the cabbage is covered by the liquid brine.

Fermented Vegetables

This recipe was originally posted on my website here: https://thehealthyrd.com/the-easiest-fermented-vegetables-recipe/ A super simple recipe for fermented vegetables that takes minutes to make. The results are tasty, fermented vegetables that you can eat after about a week of fermenting and they keep for months in the refrigerator.

Prep Time: 20 minutes.
    Equipment

- 1 Wide mouth lid and jar
- 1 small glass
- 1 Liquid measuring cup
- 1 Cutting board

Ingredients

- 2 cups filtered water
- 1.5 tbsp Himalayan, Redmond salt, or sea salt don't use iodized salt
- 3 tbsp Apple cider vinegar with the mother
- 4 cups Chopped vegetables, such as cauliflower, carrots, and onions

1. Stir the salt, filtered water, and vinegar (optional) together in a liquid measuring cup. Set aside.
2. Chop up your desired vegetables on a cutting board into bite-sized pieces.
3. In your wide-mouth mason jar, tightly pack in the vegetables until they are 1/2 inch from the top rim of the jar.
4. Pour the saltwater mixture over the top of the vegetables, making sure all the vegetables are covered in liquid completely. Leave at least 1/4 inch space at the top.
5. To keep the vegetables submerged in liquid, place a clean small glass on the top. Alternatively you can place a cabbage leaf on the top to keep the vegetables in the water. It is very important to keep the vegetables submerged so that they ferment properly.
6. Ferment the vegetables at room temperature and keep out of direct light for 5-7 days or until it has the flavor you desire. The warmer your room, the quicker they will ferment.
7. Once they reach your desired flavor, you can then store them. Cover with a wide mouth mason lid and store in the refrigerator for up to 6 months.

Fermented Rice

Fermenting rice is super easy and helps improve its health properties. It helps remove antinutrients in the grain too, making its nutrients more absorbable.

Simple Soak Method

Directions: Grab a big bowl, cover your rice with water, put a lid on, and check it in about a day. That's all you have to do. Drain off the rice water or save it for future batches. Then, cook the rice, reducing the cooking time because fermentation softens the grain.

Some research shows that baking soda may further help reduce phytic acid, an antinutrient in grains, so feel free to throw a pinch of baking soda in the mix for soaking.

Around 75 to 86 degrees Fahrenheit is optimal for rice fermentation, and this holds true with traditional methods of rice fermentation too. If your house isn't this warm, consider putting the rice in an Instant Pot and using the yogurt setting.

Be aware that if you ferment rice too long, it will become rice wine; not exactly what we are after here.

Save the soaking water each time. This will speed up the fermentation next time and reduce the anti-nutrients more quickly in subsequent fermented rice batches. Bonus: fermented brown rice cooks quickly in about 30 minutes, which makes it easier if you are busy on a weeknight.

Cultured Method

Adding yeast also helps speed up the fermentation of rice and other grains. Simply soak the rice in water with a teaspoon of yeast the day before you intend to cook the rice.

Distiller's yeast is helpful for this. I use the Red Star Dady type.

Cook the rice as you would normally but reduce the cooking time for white rice to about 8 minutes, and for brown rice, the cooking time will be about 30 minutes.

Spicy Sweet Potato Hash Browns

This dish goes nicely with poached eggs or with natural Bratwurst sausages. You can also serve it with a burger patty or sauteed chicken and greens of your choice to make a complete meal.

- 2 tbsp of coconut oil or butter
- 2 medium sweet potatoes diced evenly
- 1 small onion diced evenly
- ½ tsp ground cinnamon
- 1/2 tsp allspice (optional)
- ¼ tsp ground nutmeg
- Pinch of sea salt
- Parmesan cheese (optional)

In a pan heated to medium add two tablespoons of coconut oil, sweet potatoes, and onions. Cover and simmer for 5-7 minutes, stirring frequently. Cook until sweet potatoes are soft, then add cinnamon, allspice, and nutmeg. Top with Parmesan cheese if you wish.

Sautéed Potatoes

Total time: 15-20 minutes Servings: 3-4

- 1 lb potatoes of choice (I like Russet)

- 2 tbsp butter
- 1 tbsp oil
- 1/4 tsp Himalayan salt
- 1/2 tsp pepper
- 1 tbsp fresh sage leaves, chopped, or 1 teaspoon dried sage

1. Cut the potatoes into ½ inch cubes.
2. Add the butter and oil to a cast iron skillet over medium heat. Once warm add in the potatoes.
3. Cover the pan and cook for about 8 minutes, until they are golden on the base side.
4. Uncover the pan and flip each potato to the other side and season with sage, salt, and pepper. Cook uncovered for another 5-6 minutes, or until golden brown.

Roasted Vegetables

This is a tasty side dish that is a go-to on busy days. You can use most any vegetable or spice that you have on hand too, making this an economical dish.

- 2 cups broccoli florets
- 2 cups cauliflower florets
- 2 cups sliced baby portobello mushrooms or mushroom of choice
- 1 cup sliced carrots
- 1 red bell pepper, chopped
- 1 small yellow onion, cut into 6 wedges
- 2 tbsp olive oil

- Himalayan salt and fresh ground pepper, to taste
- 1½ tsp Italian Seasoning or herbs of choice
- ½ tsp garlic powder
- grated Parmesan cheese, for garnish (optional)
- chopped fresh parsley, for garnish (optional)

1. Preheat the oven to 425°F.
2. Line a large baking sheet with foil or parchment paper.
3. Add all the vegetables to the baking sheet.
4. Add olive oil over the veggies and mix with either a wooden spoon or just use your hands.
5. Season with salt, pepper, Italian Seasoning, and garlic powder; gently toss until thoroughly combined.
6. Arrange all the veggies in a single layer.
7. Bake for 15 to 20 minutes, stirring halfway through cooking. You want to roast the veggies until fork tender and lightly browned.
8. Remove from the oven.
9. Garnish with Parmesan cheese and parsley and serve.

Sweet Potato Fries Air Fryer Style

This super easy side goes well with just about any dish. You can also use Russet potatoes in this recipe instead, but you may need to increase the cooking time to get them crispy.

Serves: 2-3 Total time: 15-20 minutes

- 1 pound sweet potatoes

- 1 tbsp extra-virgin olive oil
- 1/4 tsp garlic powder
- 1/3 tsp salt , I used pink Himalayan salt, adjust to taste
- 1/8 tsp black pepper, freshly cracked, adjust to taste

Cube the sweet potatoes into 1/2-inch pieces. Transfer the sweet potatoes to a bowl. Add the oil and seasonings. Toss them well, so they are all coated with the seasoning. Preheat the air fryer to 400°F. Add the seasoned sweet potatoes to the air fryer and spread them in a single layer, cooking in batches if needed. Air fry for 10-12 minutes or until desired crispiness.

For the oven instead:

Preheat the oven to 425°F. Transfer the sweet potatoes to a large sheet pan. You can also add olive oil and seasonings to the sheet pan. Spread evenly so they do not overlap. Cook for 25-30 minutes. Flip every 10-15 minutes for even cooking.

Perfect Sauteed Broccoli

Raw broccoli is the healthiest for hormones, but can be too bitter for some people. Sauteing broccoli retains many of the hormone-balancing nutrients, but you should cook these for as short of a period as possible to get the most benefits.

Total Time: 15 Minutes Servings: 4

- 1 large head of broccoli
- 2 Tbsp. extra-virgin olive oil or butter
- ½ tsp. kosher salt
- ¼ tsp. freshly ground black pepper

Chapter 9

- 1 to 2 tsp. fresh lemon juice
- ¼ tsp red pepper flakes (optional)

Cut the head of broccoli into bite-sized pieces. Heat the olive oil or butter in a large skillet. Once oil is shimmering, add broccoli and cook on medium heat for about 5 to 7 minutes total, stirring frequently to avoid burning. Season with salt, pepper, lemon juice, and red pepper flakes if using.

Section 3: Main Dishes

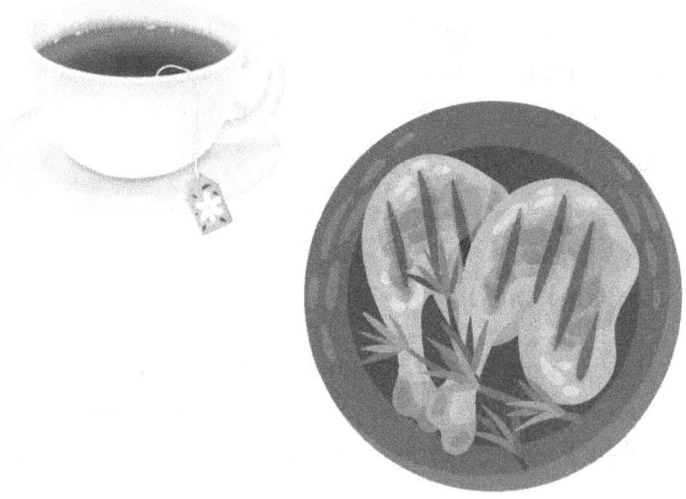

Here are 14 main dish recipes, some of which have been in my kitchen for my whole life. Cooking these at home can be rewarding in so many ways!

Versatile Chicken Vegetable Soup

Soups are truly indispensable for a healthy lifestyle and the most comforting of all is a simple chicken and vegetable soup made with nourishing ingredients. You can use any vegetables you like but these are ones I suggest in this recipe.

Prep time: 10 minutes Cook time: 40 minutes Serves: 4-6

- 2 tbsp extra-virgin olive oil
- 1 ¼ lbs. chicken
- Himalayan salt/Pepper
- 3 tbspbutter
- 1 white onion, diced
- ¾ cup carrots, sliced
- 2 ribs celery, sliced
- 3 cloves garlic, minced
- 1 tsp hot sauce (optional)
- 7 cups chicken bone broth
- 2 tsp Better than Bouillon vegetable base
- 1 ½ cups frozen mixed vegetables of your choice
- Seasonings
- 1 tsp dried sage
- 1 tspof each: dried basil, oregano, mustard powder
- ¼ tsp pepper

1. Pat chicken dry and season with salt/pepper. Heat olive oil in a 4.5-quart soup pot over medium high heat. Add the chicken and sear on each side for about 3 minutes, until a golden crust develops.

2. Remove the chicken and set aside. Let it rest for 10 minutes, then dice or shred.
3. Melt butter in the same pot over medium heat.
4. Add the onions, carrots, and celery and soften for 5 minutes, scraping the bottom of the pan to loosen any bits of chicken left on the bottom of the pan.
5. Add the garlic, hot sauce, vegetable base, Worcestershire sauce, and seasonings. Stir to combine.
6. Add the chicken broth. Bring to a boil, then reduce to a simmer. Add the chicken back to the soup along with any juice from the plate and simmer, uncovered, for 15 minutes.
7. Add the frozen vegetables. Cover partially and simmer for 10-15 more minutes.

Healthy Chicken Nuggets

A common misconception is that you can't use olive oil to fry with. This is not true if you use extra virgin olive oil. The antioxidants in this oil protect it from oxidation and even convey some important nutrients to this dish. Popular with kids and adults alike, chicken nuggets can be a healthy option if made with care like this recipe. Adapted from Alex Snodgrass's *Defined Dish Cookbook*.

Marinate time: 2 hours Prep time: 15 minutes Cook time: 5 minutes.

- 1 ½ pounds of boneless, skinless chicken breasts
- ½ cup dill pickle juice or ¼ cup rice vinegar and ½ teaspoon salt
- 2 eggs, whisked with 1 tbsp water
- ½ cup tapioca or arrowroot starch
- ½ cup almond flour

- 1 tsp garlic powder
- 1 tsp onion powder
- 1 tsp paprika
- ⅛ tsp cayenne pepper (optional)
- 1 ½ tsp Himalayan salt
- ½ tsp black pepper
- ½ cup extra virgin olive oil
- Dipping sauce of choice (try with the Burger Bowl sauce on page 262 if you wish)

1. Pound the chicken breasts, between two layers of parchment paper, until about ¼-inch thick. Cut the chicken into pieces that are chicken nugget size, about 2 inches big.
2. Combine the chicken with the pickle juice and marinate for 2 or more hours.
3. Drain off the pickle juice. Add the egg mixture to a bowl and in a separate bowl, combine the almond flour and tapioca flour along with the garlic powder, onion powder, paprika, cayenne pepper, black pepper, and salt and salt.
4. Dredge the chicken as follows: dip the chicken in the egg combination, dipping each piece in the mixture and setting aside. Next, dredge each piece of chicken in the flour mixture.
5. Using a Dutch oven or deep skillet, heat the olive oil over medium heat. Cook chicken in hot oil in batches where the chicken isn't touching in the pan and has plenty of room to crisp up. This will take several batches. Cook for about 3 minutes on the first side or until nice and brown and then flip for about 1-2 minutes on the other side to be nice and crispy.

Dip in your favorite sauce.

Chapter 9

Savory Slow-Cooker Pepper Steak

This is a favorite of mine from my childhood. So savory and tender and nutrient-rich for your hormone balance as a bonus!

Total Time: 3 hrs. 30 mins Servings: 6

- 2 pounds beef sirloin, cut into 2-inch strips
- ¾ tsp garlic powder, or to taste
- 3 tsp extra virgin olive oil
- 1 tsp beef base
- ¼ cup hot water
- 2 tbsp cassava flour or 1 tablespoon cornstarch
- ½ cup chopped onion
- 2 large green bell peppers, roughly chopped
- 1 (14.5 ounce) can stewed tomatoes, with liquid
- 3 tbsp coconut aminos
- 1/4 tsp Himalayan salt

1. Sprinkle beef with garlic powder. Heat olive oil in a large skillet over medium heat and sear beef strips, about 5 minutes per side. If you have an Instant Pot, you can sauté it there. Transfer to a slow cooker if using a slow cooker.
2. Mix beef base with hot water in a separate container until dissolved, then mix in cassava flour or cornstarch until dissolved.
3. Pour into the slow cooker with beef strips. Stir in onion, green peppers, stewed tomatoes, coconut aminos, and salt.
4. Cover, and cook on High for 3 to 4 hours, or on Low for 6 to 8 hours.

Super Quick Sausage and Vegetables

You can add any vegetable that you like to the dish, and I encourage you to use what you have on hand. Beets are also great here if you enjoy beets. You don't even have to peel them; simply dice up the beets into small pieces because they take a bit longer to cook than other vegetables.

Total time: 30 minutes Servings: 4-6

- 12-16 ounces organic sausage, about 3 cups
- 2 cups sweet potato, diced into 1/2" cubes
- 2 cups Brussels sprouts coarsely chopped
- 1 onion coarsely chopped
- 1 red bell pepper, coarsely chopped
- 2 tbsp extra-virgin olive oil
- 1 tbsp spice blend of your choice
- ½ tsp salt
- ½ tsp black pepper

1. Preheat oven to 400F. Slice the sausage into 1–2-inch rounds. Dice the sweet potatoes into small 1/2' cubes.
2. Add the sausage, veggies, and minced garlic to a large baking sheet. Drizzle with olive oil and sprinkle with your favorite spice blend. Add salt and pepper if you wish. Toss veggies with your hands until they are fully combined and coated with olive oil and spices.
3. Bake for 20 minutes, flipping halfway. Enjoy with fermented rice or the side of your choice.

Chapter 9

Liver, Vodka, and Onions

You really should try this recipe even if you are squeamish about liver; it is tender like a filet mignon. The key is that buttermilk reduces any heavy liver taste. The generous number of onions and garlic along with the vodka complement the liver quite well. Try taking a bit of sauteed onions with each bite of liver if you still don't enjoy the flavor of the meat. But I feel like most liver skeptics can learn to appreciate eating liver by making this dish. The vodka mostly cooks off but you can certainly substitute chicken broth or beef broth for the vodka if you want to omit it.

Marinate time: 2 hours Prep time: 10 minutes Cook time: 20 minutes

- 1 cups buttermilk
- 3 tbsp (45 ml) extra-virgin olive oil or butter
- 2 garlic cloves, minced
- ¾ pound beef liver, sliced into strips
- Salt and black pepper to taste
- 2 tbsp butter
- 2 large onions, thinly sliced
- 1/4 cup vodka
- Fresh parsley, chopped

- To reduce the strong taste of the meat, place the liver in a bowl and cover with buttermilk. Refrigerate for up to 2 hours. Then remove the liver from the liquid and pat dry.
- Heat a large cast-iron skillet over medium to medium-high heat. Add the olive oil and heat. Add garlic and saute until fragrant, stirring constantly to avoid burning, about 1 – 2 minutes. Then add the liver strips and fry until crispy browned on both sides. Season with salt and

pepper to taste. Remove the liver from the skillet with a slotted spoon and set it aside on a plate or bowl.
- Add the butter to the same skillet. Saute the sliced onions until translucent and fragrant about 8 minutes. Add the liver back to the skillet and add the vodka. Let the vodka reduce for 2 – 3 minutes.
- Garnish with fresh parsley and serve warm.

Honey-Garlic Shrimp and Broccoli

This super simple recipe features hormone-balancing broccoli and shrimp. Unlike other stir-fry recipes, this features more protein to support the building blocks of hormones and more omega 3's from shrimp for healthy cell membranes. And unlike many people think, raw honey is rich in enzymes and prebiotics that support healthy gut and hormone health as well as immunity. Serve with cauliflower rice or fermented rice and a green salad if you wish.

Prep time: 10 minutes Cook time: 15 minutes Total time: 25 minutes 4 servings

- 4 tbsp extra-virgin olive oil, divided
- 4 cloves garlic, sliced, divided, about 2 ½ tbsp
- 4 cups small broccoli florets
- ½ tsp Himalayan salt
- ½ tsp ground pepper, divided
- 2 pounds peeled and deveined medium-sized raw shrimp (20-30 count)
- 4-5 tbsp lemon juice, plus more to taste if you wish
- ¼ cup local raw honey
- Pinch of red pepper flakes (optional)

Heat 2 tablespoons of oil in a large pot over medium heat. Add half the garlic and cook until beginning to brown, about 1 minute. Add broccoli, ½ teaspoon salt and 1/4 teaspoon pepper. Cover and cook, stirring once or twice until the vegetables are crisp-tender, about 2 to 4 minutes. Remove the broccoli from the pan.

Increase the heat to medium-high and add the remaining 1 tablespoon oil to the pot. Add the remaining garlic and cook until beginning to brown, about 1 minute. Add half of the shrimp and the remaining pepper. Cook, stirring, until the shrimp are just cooked through and turned pink, about 3-5 minutes. Remove the shrimp from the pan and cook the remaining shrimp for another 3-5 minutes until pink. Return the broccoli mixture to the pot along with lemon juice, honey, and red pepper flakes (if using). Stir to combine and heat through.

*Note: Add about 1 teaspoon lemon zest to this dish for an even more intense lemon flavor.

Creamy Chicken with Mushrooms

Many people shy away from saturated fats, but this shirking of saturated fats can spell disaster for hormones. There is also no real evidence that avoiding saturated fats is protective for the heart either especially for women of reproductive age. This recipe contains butter and cream to support hormone production in the body. For people who don't tolerate dairy, simply use more olive oil instead of butter and use unsweetened coconut cream instead of heavy cream. You can use button mushrooms, but if you can get your hands on Lion's mane mushrooms, I highly encourage you to use these because they are extra delicious and are calming to the brain, aka an adaptogen for hormones.

- 4 chicken cutlets, patted dry
- Salt and pepper
- 2 tbsp extra-virgin olive oil
- Gluten free flour, for dredging
- 1 tbsp butter
- 2 green onions, thinly sliced
- 8 ounces mushrooms (any edible kind you like), sliced, preferably Lion's mane mushrooms
- 1 1/4 cups organic chicken bone broth
- 3/4 cup organic heavy cream

Preheat the oven to 200 degrees F. Heat a large skillet with 1 tablespoon olive oil over medium-high heat. Season the chicken with salt and pepper, then dredge 2 chicken cutlets in flour, shake off any excess, and place them in the skillet. Cook the chicken until golden, about 1 1/2 minutes per side and then transfer to a baking dish. Repeat with the remaining 1 tablespoon oil and the other 2 chicken cutlets. Cover the dish loosely with foil; place in a warming oven while you prepare the vegetables.

Add the butter to the hot skillet, then add the scallions and mushrooms; cook, stirring occasionally, until the mushrooms brown, about 4 minutes. Pour in the broth and bring to a boil, scraping up any browned bits with a wooden spoon. Cook until the liquid is reduced by half, about 3 minutes. Add the cream and boil until the sauce thickens slightly, 3 to 4 more minutes. Stir in the snap peas and heat through, season with salt and pepper. Serve the chicken topped with the creamy mushrooms.

Pesto Salmon with Tomatoes

This sheet pan pesto salmon with tomatoes is perfect for fast, healthy dinners. The salmon is tender and flaky, and the pesto makes it taste fresh!

Chapter 9

I highly recommend that you make your own pesto. Store-bought pesto almost always uses cheap and unhealthy oils in their products.

Total time: 45 minutes Servings: 4 servings

- 4 (6-ounce) salmon filets, skin on
- 1/2 tsp Himalayan salt divided, plus additional for serving
- 1/2 tsp ground black pepper divided
- 6 tsp prepared basil pesto divided (see recipe below)
- 2 pints cherry or grape tomatoes left whole
- 1 small red onion thinly sliced
- Squeeze of fresh lemon juice for serving
- Chopped fresh basil optional for serving

Place a rack in the center of your oven and preheat the oven to 400 degrees F. Generously coat a large, rimmed baking sheet with nonstick spray. Place the cherry tomatoes and red onion in a large bowl. Add 2 tablespoons of pesto, 1/4 teaspoon salt, and ¼ teaspoon black pepper. Toss to coat, then spread into a single layer on the prepared baking sheet. Bake the tomatoes and onion for 10 minutes, then remove from the oven and with a spatula, stir them around a little to promote even cooking, then return to the oven for 10 additional minutes. Meanwhile, pat the salmon filets dry. Sprinkle with 1/4 teaspoon salt and 1/4 teaspoon black pepper. Spread 1 tablespoon of the remaining pesto over each fillet. Rub the pesto on with your fingers or the back of a small spoon as needed. Make sure each filet is completely covered in pesto. Remove the sheet pan from the oven and move the tomatoes and onions to the outsides to make space for the salmon in the center. Arrange the salmon filets down the center of the baking sheet, skin-side down. Return the pan to the oven and bake the pesto salmon until the fish flakes easily with a fork and reaches an internal temperature of 145 degrees F, about 16 to 20 minutes. Sprinkle the salmon with a pinch of additional salt and squeeze lemon over the top. Top with fresh basil as desired.

Note: The cooking time will vary based upon the thickness of your salmon. Thicker (2-inch-plus) slices will need several extra minutes, while thinner slices may cook more quickly.

Homemade Pesto

Most recipes call for pine nuts, but they are quite expensive, and walnuts taste as good or better than pine nuts in this recipe. This economical version fits any budget, and the leftovers can be to finish chicken, meats, and vegetables to make any dish more tasty.

Prep time: 2 minutes Total time: 5 minutes

- 2 cups fresh basil leaves
- 1/3 cup walnuts
- 2-3 garlic cloves
- ½-¾ cup extra-virgin olive oil
- 1/2 cup freshly grated Parmesan cheese

1. Combine basil, walnuts, and garlic in the bowl of a food processor or blender. Chop until finely chopped.
2. Add olive oil slowly into the food processor as it is running until pesto is at your desired consistency. I prefer more olive oil.
3. Add the Parmesan cheese and process until mixed well.

Air Fryer Salmon Rice Bowl

This dish makes a great dish any time of the year and is an easy way to fit in lots of hormone-healthy foods like salmon and ginger.

- 16 ounces wild salmon
- 1 tbsp extra-virgin olive oil
- 1 cup Basmati or another rice-make fermented if possible, recipe on page 241
- 2 cups water
- ¼ cup avocado mayonnaise
- 2 tsp Sriracha hot sauce
- 1 tbsp coconut aminos
- 1 ½ tsp freshly grated ginger
- ¼ tsp crushed red pepper (optional)
- 1 ripe avocado, sliced
- 1 cup chopped, peeled cucumber
- 1 cup chopped red cabbage
- 12 (4 inch) sheets nori (roasted seaweed)

1. Preheat the air fryer to 400ºF.
2. Coat the salmon with oil. Air fry the salmon until the salmon flakes easily with a fork, about 10 minutes for a thinner filet and 20 minutes for a thicker salmon filet.
3. Meanwhile, combine rice and water in a small saucepan; cook 5 minutes for fermentation and 15 minutes for white rice.
4. Mix mayonnaise and Sriracha (optional) in a small bowl; set aside. Whisk coconut aminos, ginger, crushed red pepper and salt in another small bowl; set aside.
5. Divide the rice between 3 bowls. Top with salmon, avocado, cucumber, and nori. Drizzle with the tamari mixture and the mayonnaise mixture. Mix the bowls, if desired, and serve with nori.

Butter Chicken

For years, this recipe has been a family favorite. It is great for leftovers and has a more mellow flavor than many butter chicken recipes. I like to grind the coriander and cumin from whole seeds because it gives a better flavor than pre-ground, but you can always use ground spices in a pinch.

For the marinated chicken:

- 2 pounds of boneless and skinless chicken thighs or breasts cut into bite-sized pieces
- 1/2 cup plain whole milk yogurt
- 1 1/2 tbsp minced garlic
- 1 tbsp finely grated ginger, peel on
- 2 tsp garam masala
- 1 tsp turmeric
- 1 tsp freshly ground cumin
- 1 tsp of Himalayan salt

For the sauce:

- 2 tbsp olive oil
- 2 tbsp butter
- 1 large onion, sliced or chopped
- 1 1/2 tbsp garlic, minced
- 1 tbsp finely grated ginger, peel on
- 1 1/2 tsp freshly ground cumin
- 1 1/2 tsp garam masala
- 1 tsp freshly ground coriander
- 14 oz (400 g) crushed tomatoes or tomato sauce

- 1 1/4 tsp salt (optional)
- 1 cup of organic heavy whipping cream
- Cilantro (optional)

1. In a bowl, combine chicken with all of the ingredients for the chicken marinade; let marinate for 30 minutes to an hour.
2. Heat olive oil in a large skillet or pot over medium-high heat. When sizzling, add chicken pieces in batches of two or three, making sure not to crowd the pan. Fry until browned for only 3 minutes on each side. Set aside and keep warm.
3. Heat butter or ghee in the same pan. Fry the onions until they start to sweat (about 6 minutes) while scraping up any browned bits stuck on the bottom of the pan.
4. Add garlic and ginger and sauté for 1 minute until fragrant, then add ground coriander, cumin and garam masala. Let cook for about 20 seconds until fragrant, while stirring occasionally.
5. Add crushed tomatoes, chili powder, and salt. Let simmer for about 10-15 minutes, stirring occasionally until sauce thickens and becomes a deep brown, red color.
6. Stir the cream into the sauce. Add the chicken with juices back into the pan and cook for an additional 8-10 minutes until chicken is cooked through and the sauce is thick and bubbling.
7. Garnish with chopped cilantro and serve with rice or potatoes if you wish.

Meatballs with Nourishing Beef Liver

Making meatballs is rewarding and extra nutritious because they contain liver. I designed this recipe to be very big so that you can freeze 2/3rds of them or as many as you want for easy weeknight meals later.

Total time: 40 minutes Makes about 40 meatballs

- 2 tsp onion powder
- 2 tsp garlic powder
- 2 tsp chili flakes (optional but recommended)
- 1 tbsp oregano
- 3 lbs. grass fed ground beef
- 1.5 lb. grass fed beef liver or organic chicken liver
- 1 ¼ cup gluten free Panko breadcrumbs
- 1 tsp Himalayan salt

1. Preheat the oven to 400 degrees F.
2. Grind the chicken liver in a food processor or blender by pulsing it a few times. Place the ground beef in a bowl. Add the liver and the rest of the ingredients, mixing thoroughly with your hands to combine evenly.
3. Form into meatballs using an ice cream scoop or large spoon.
4. Bake for 30 mins or until browned at 400 degrees F.
5. Serve with gravy or sauce of your choice.
6. Freeze any extra meatballs for a later date.

Burger Bowls

I like to serve these with air fryer homemade Air Fryer Sweet Potato fries or russet potato fries (see recipe included on page 244).

Makes 2-3 salads

- 1 lb. grass fed ground beef

- ½ lb. ground chicken or beef liver
- Worcestershire sauce
- homemade seasoned salt and pepper
- 2-3 heads romaine lettuce, chopped
- 1 red onion, thinly sliced
- 1 Roma tomato, chopped (can use cherry, grape, or vine-ripened tomatoes)
- 1/2 cup chopped dill pickles

For the Special Sauce Salad Dressing:

- 1 cup avocado mayonnaise
- 2 tbsp minced pickles
- 2 tbsp minced white onion
- ⅛ tsp cayenne pepper (optional)
- 1 tbsp distilled white vinegar
- 1 tbsp honey

- For the Special Sauce Salad Dressing: Add ingredients to a bowl then whisk to combine. Can be done several days ahead of time.
- Heat a large skillet over medium-high heat then add the ground beef and ground liver.
- Let the beef cook undisturbed until the bottom is golden brown then add a few shakes of Worcestershire sauce, season with homemade seasoned salt and pepper, and continue to saute until cooked through.
- Scoop onto a paper towel lined plate to drain and cool slightly. Once slightly cooled, divvy lettuce between plates or bowls then tops with the cooked ground beef, red onion, tomatoes, and dill pickles.
- Drizzle with Special Sauce Salad Dressing then serve.

Section 4: Cravings

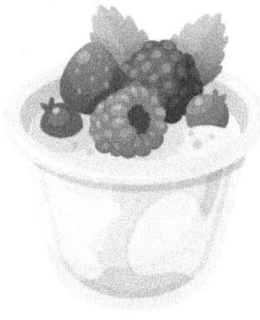

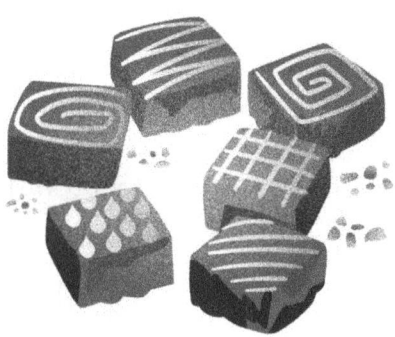

While sweets aren't often on the menu for best period health, there are some ways to get a healthy taste of sweetness in your life on occasion. Here are a few favorite ways that I like to satisfy my sweet tooth.

Healthy Honey Lemonade/Limeade

When I converted my diet to no-added-sugar and eliminated all the junk for the most part, I learned that I craved citrus in a big way. In honor of these cravings, I give you my favorite way to have lemonade with no guilt. With only 8 grams of sugar, this recipe hits just right when the weather warms up. Compare this to an average soda with over 45 grams of sugar and you can feel pretty good about this drink.

- Juice of ½ of lemon or a whole lime
- Zest of ½ of lemon or lime (optional but recommended)
- 1 heaping tsp local raw honey
- Filtered water

Mix the lemon juice, honey, and zest. Let it sit until dissolved, about 5 minutes. Mix in water and ice, then serve.

Wholesome Chocolates

Let's face it; we all love chocolate and sometimes hormones make the desire for this treat irresistible. You can make chocolate healthy if you use a sweetener like honey that happens to be good for hormones and the immune system.

- 1/2 cup organic cocoa butter or coconut oil
- ⅓ cup organic cacao powder, such as Terrasoil brand (ethically sourced). You can use cocoa powder if you can't find it.
- 2 tbsp local raw honey
- 1 tsp vanilla extract

Melt cocoa butter or coconut oil in a double boiler. Remove from heat and stir with a spoon or spatula for 2 minutes. Transfer to a room temperature glass bowl. Stir for 2 minutes or until mixture is 90° Fahrenheit. Mix in cacao or cocoa powder and honey. Stir well. Add vanilla extract and stir with a whisk until smooth. Pour into chocolate mold and allow to sit at room temperature until hardened. If you don't have a mold, you can use a cookie sheet that has parchment paper on it to harden the chocolate and then break it up into pieces from there. Remove chocolate from mold or cookie sheet and store at room temperature. If your house is warm you may want to keep the chocolate in the refrigerator.

Berry-Yogurt "Dessert"

I often make a variation of this depending on what flavor profile I want. For example, I will often use lemon zest because I love lemon, but cinnamon is delicious too. If you add collagen to this, it helps boost your skin health and helps support better bone density and all women can stand a bit more of that.

Total time: 2 minutes Servings: 1

- 1 tsp Ceylon cinnamon or 1 teaspoon lemon zest
- 1 cup plain organic whole milk yogurt
- ⅓ cup berries of choice
- 1 tsp honey (optional)
- 1 scoop collagen powder (optional but encouraged)

Mix all of the ingredients together and serve.

High Protein "Shake"

Shakes aren't usually on the menu when you are trying to get your hormones healthy. But a whey protein shake is a totally different ball game. It can really help improve your hormones indirectly by increasing fullness, helping prevent overeating of carbs, and helping provide building blocks for hormones. Did you know that whey protein is one of the best ways to help increase GLP1? This is the hormone that the new weight loss drugs target, only whey protein does so safely, albeit more mildly. I'm often too lazy to drag out the blender so I sip on my vanilla whey protein with just plain water. But to make it more shake-like, you can throw it in the blender with some ice and fruit.

- 1 large scoop grass-fed whey protein powder (no fake sugars)
- Ice
- ½ tsp Ceylon cinnamon or ground cardamom
- ½ banana or other fruit of choice (optional)
- 1 cup of water

Blend all of these together and serve.

Ten

Chapter 10

Conclusion

Period issues affect the majority of women and yet conventional medications only touch the surface of menstrual concerns while often ignoring the deep root causes of these period maladies. Fortunately you don't have to live with these constant issues most of the time if you are able to incorporate a more holistic way of living as reviewed throughout this book.

I sincerely hope that some of the strategies that I provided helps you improve your hormonal health and overall health. Keep in mind that we are all unique. We aren't built from a cookie cutter so it may take exploring a number of natural lifestyle changes to make you feel your best. You also may find that using a multi-faceted approach works better than a single-step approach. For example, if you have perimenopausal symptoms, it may be best to follow meal planning strategies in Chapter 8 and incorporate multiple herbs like black cohosh, vitex, turmeric, and DHEA along with nutrient supplements as described in Chapter 4.

Chapter 10

Using traditional healing that is research-supported as reviewed throughout this text is truly empowering-at least it has been for me and the women that I know. Your learning shouldn't stop here, however. I encourage you to use this book as a reference and continue to explore the ongoing research that is found in the National Library of Medicine and even find online forums for your specific period concerns. While these aren't authoritative necessarily, it may spark an area of research that you can then verify through the Library of Medicine. Discuss these with your provider. Keep asking questions until you get answers that resonate with how you want to be cared for.

When it comes to your hormonal health and period health, be curious, always keep learning, and use a risk-benefit assessment for each step you take along the way. And remember, finding a supportive healthcare provider to address your issues in an open-minded way is perhaps the most powerful thing you can do for your overall health. This can take some shopping around because of the current dogmatic ways of thinking in medicine. I suggest that you find a reputable naturopath along with a holistically-trained physician. Using the Institute for Functional Medicine website can help you find a provider like this in your area.

Last but not least, I encourage you to spread the word about this book and share it with your loved ones. Odds are, they may be suffering in silence too. Or they may have a loved one that is struggling with menstrual issues as well.

Eleven

Chapter 11

Glossary

- **Adaptogen herbs**: Herbs and some kinds of mushrooms that help the body adapt to stress.
- **Agonist:** A compound that activates a cell response.
- **Analgesic:** Anything that dampens or reduces pain.
- **Antibodies**: Proteins in the body that play a role in immunity by finding foreign particles and mounting an immune response. Foods can be a source of antibodies and can cause inflammation if a person is reactive to them.
- **Antioxidants**: Substances that reduce oxidative damage in the body.
- **Antiviral**: A substance that helps reduce viral infections.
- **ApoE4 genotype:** A type of gene variant that increases the risk of Alzheimer's disease and cardiovascular disease.
- **Aromatase**: an enzyme that converts testosterone to estrogen.
- **Ayurvedic**: A type of traditional medicine used in India and other parts of the world. This type of medicine seeks to create balance in the body.

- **Beta-glucuronidase**: An enzyme that activates estrogen. It has other roles in the body such as the breakdown of carbohydrates. Too much beta-glucuronidase can lead to hormonal imbalance.
- **Bioavailable**: A nutrient or compound that absorbs and is used by the body easily.
- **Bioidentical**: Means that a compound is identical to ones found in the human body.
- **Cardioprotective**: Anything that helps prevent health issues with the heart and blood vessels.
- **Cervical dysplasia**: Cells on the cervix that aren't normal cells.
- **Cofactor**: A factor involved in making an enzyme active in the body. These are often vitamins, antioxidants, amino acids, and minerals.
- **Compounds**: Substances formed from the union of two separate substances.
- **Cortisol steal**: A shift in hormones where cortisol is elevated for prolonged periods and this results in the body making more cortisol and stealing from other hormones like estrogen, progesterone, and testosterone. This is often due to stress and lack of nutrients.
- **DHEA** (Dehydroepiandrosterone): Is a hormone that is the parent hormone to estrogen, progesterone, and testosterone. It also has its own functions, including regulation of insulin sensitivity and immunity. It is also protective for nerve cells.
- **Diuretic**: A substance that promotes an increase in urine production.
- **Dopamine**: A type of nerve chemical naturally made in the body that promotes feelings of pleasure, motivation, and happiness.
- **Dysmenorrhea**: is pain during the menstrual cycle.
- **Endocannabinoid system:** A system in the body that regulates balance through messages between cells involved in mood, appetite, pain, immunity, and more.
- **Endometriosis** A condition where uterine tissue grows outside the uterus, such as in the bladder, bowel, or ovaries. This condition causes a lot of pain especially in the second half of the menstrual cycle.
- **Endometrial ablation:** A procedure that destroys the uterine tissue

by either heat or cold.
- **Estrogen dominance**: Occurs when estrogen levels are higher in proportion to other hormones in the body like progesterone. It is linked to health conditions like heavy periods, increased cancer risk and other diseases like blood clots.
- **Fibroids**: Non-cancerous tumors that grow in and around the uterus.
- **Fibromyalgia:** Is a pain and fatigue syndrome often related to excess toxins and inadequate nutrients.
- **Genitourinary symptoms**: Symptoms affecting the urinary tract and genital organs in women and are often tied to menopause. These symptoms can include vaginal dryness, vaginal thinning, urinary frequency, urinary tract infections, and pain during sexual activity.
- **Goitrogen**: a substance that interferes with thyroid function and/or thyroid structure.
- **Good Manufacturing Practices**: A set of guidelines that ensure the quality and safety of products, particularly in the world of supplements. It involves inspections of facilities for contaminants, safety, quality, and purity.
- **Gut epithelial cells:** Protective cells in the gut lining but are only one cell thick. This makes them vulnerable to toxins and the foods we eat. They are central to immune function, nutrient absorption, and form a physical barrier between the gut and the rest of the body.
- **Hashimoto's thyroiditis**: A type of autoimmune thyroid disease where the body mistakenly attacks its own thyroid tissue. This condition can be triggered or worsened by some foods and food sensitivities.
- **Homocysteine:** A normal substance in the blood that can become excessive because of a lack of vitamins or a lack of methyl compounds in the body.
- **Hysterectomy**: A type of surgery to remove the uterus.
- **Ibuprofen**: A non-steroidal anti-inflammatory pain medication that is over-the-counter. While it helps reduce pain, it comes with a lot of side effects if used frequently, such as gastrointestinal distress, bleeding, kidney issues, and more.

- **Inflammation**: A necessary response to an injury or stress in the body that results in symptoms of pain, redness, swelling, and heat. Long-term inflammation due to modern lifestyles, however, is linked to increased risk of most diseases today.
- **Insulin resistance**: Is when the body doesn't respond to insulin well because of excess carbohydrates, increased belly fat, lack of exercise, lack of nutrients, and certain medications.
- **Intermittent fasting**: Is done by eating and fasting in defined periods of time and this is done to improve metabolic health.
- **Insulin receptor**: A place on cells that receive signals from insulin.
- **Ketogenic diet**: A diet that is low in carbohydrates, moderate in proteins, and higher in fats. This type of diet leads to ketosis, which aids in weight loss, diabetes management, and neurological conditions for some people.
- **Luteal cells**: Cells where progesterone is made in the body.
- **Luteal phase**: The phase where progesterone production is increased in order to prepare the uterus for pregnancy or for the next menstrual period.
- **Mastalgia**: breast pain.
- **Metabolic syndrome**: A syndrome related to processed foods that leads to increased abdominal fat, high blood pressure, Type 2 diabetes, abnormal blood fats, heart disease, and cancer risk.
- **Metabolites**: compounds that are intermediates in metabolism of nutrients or other compounds.
- **Metformin**: A prescription medication used to reduce sugar absorption and improve insulin sensitivity. However, it reduces the absorption of vitamin B12 and has multiple digestive side effects.
- **Microbiome**: Your body's collection of living bacteria, viruses, and fungi that live within the digestive tract and skin that send signals throughout the whole body and mind.
- **Mitochondria**: The energy-producing parts of each cell.
- **Mittelschmerz**: Pain related to ovulation or the second half of the menstrual phase that can last for many days.

- **Non-steroidal anti-inflammatory medications:** Over-the-counter and prescription drugs that are used to decrease inflammation, but carry a host of side effects.
- **Oxalates:** Natural compounds in foods and made by the body that cause inflammation and pain in some people.
- **Ovarian cysts**: Fluid-filled sacs in the ovaries that are common but can cause significant pain if they are large or caused by endometriosis.
- **Neurotransmitters**: Natural chemical signals that allow nerves to communicate with each other.
- **Nitric oxide**: a compound that causes blood vessels to dilate and decreases blood pressure.
- **Norepinephrine**: Is both a hormone and a neurotransmitter which is involved in the stress response in the body, pain regulation, and mood regulation.
- **Parasympathetic**: is the nervous system response that promotes relaxation and digestion.
- **Phytates**: compounds found in plants, especially grains, that bind nutrients, especially minerals like zinc and calcium, making them unavailable for absorption.
- **Phytoestrogens**: Plant compounds that have similar structures to estrogen but by binding estrogen receptors often have anti-estrogen effects in the body. At times, they can also have estrogenic effects in the body too.
- **Polycystic ovarian syndrome**: A condition with multiple ovarian cysts, menstrual cycle irregularities, and an increase in male hormones and insulin.
- **PPARγ** (peroxisome proliferator-activated receptor gamma): Helps regulate sugar and fat metabolism and also has anti-inflammatory effects in the body.
- **Preclinical:** A type of study that is conducted in cells or in animals and is not done in humans.
- **Probiotics**: Beneficial, living microorganisms.
- **Processed foods**: Foods that have undergone significant processing

in a factory, such as frozen meals, snacks, fast foods, sugary beverages, baked goods, and more. This processing often destroys nutrients and makes foods less healthy than minimally processed foods.
- **Prohormone**: An inactive substance that undergoes modification in the body to make a hormone.
- **Psychoactive**: A substance that can affect the mind.
- **Reuptake:** Is when chemical messengers are reabsorbed into the neuron. Medications are used to reduce reuptake so that more chemical messengers are available in parts of the nervous system.
- **Selective estrogen receptor modulator:** A compound that mimics the beneficial effects of estrogen while minimizing its harmful effects on reproductive tissue.
- **Side benefits**: Benefits beyond the expected benefits often related to herbs and natural compounds.
- **Steroid hormones**: Hormones in the body made from cholesterol. This includes estrogen, progesterone, testosterone, cortisol, and DHEA.
- **Sulforaphane**: A natural antioxidant found in cruciferous vegetables that naturally dampen inflammation.
- **Synergism**: Is when two or more things are combined and have a greater effect than the sum of its parts.
- **Toxin**: Any poisonous or unhealthy substance that enters the body.
- **Vasomotor symptoms**: Are caused by sudden constriction or dilation of the blood vessels that leads to symptoms of hot flashes, night sweats, and/or cold chills.

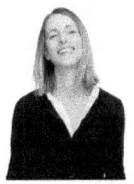

About the Author

Heidi Moretti, MS, RD, is a registered dietitian at Fresenius Medical Care and owns The Healthy RD LLC, a blog and resource for people looking for natural and scientifically proven remedies for health issues. She received post-graduate school training through the Institute for Functional Medicine and is constantly using the National Library of Medicine to uncover natural medicines research. She is the author of the bestselling book Gut Fix, The Whole Body Guide to Gut Health and The Elimination Diet Journal. She has published numerous clinical research studies as the principal investigator for these studies, including:

"Vitamin D3 repletion versus placebo as adjunctive treatment of heart failure patient quality of life and hormonal indices: a randomized, double-blind, placebo-controlled trial."

"Biotin Deficiency as a target for treating restless legs syndrome in chronic dialysis patients."

"Effects of protein supplementation in chronic hemodialysis and peritoneal dialysis patients."

"Prevalence of low albumin, suboptimal energy, and muscle stores in Asian dialysis patients."

Additionally, she worked for over twenty years at Providence Saint Patrick Hospital in Missoula, where she honed her clinical skills and continued to find ways to add functional medicine into a conventional world.

You can connect with me on:
- https://thehealthyrd.com
- https://twitter.com/HeidiHmoretti

Also by Heidi Moretti

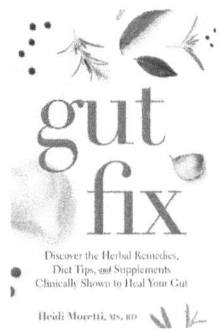

Gut Fix

Gut Fix is a refreshing and unique guide that specifically walks you through safe dietary supplements and diet strategies to try when you have been cleared to do so by your healthcare provider. This book helps you learn about the proper use of these supplements and how they may help many of the symptoms you may be having.

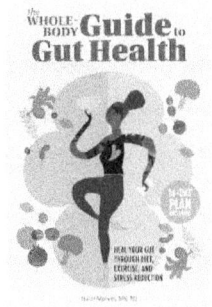

The Whole Body Guide to Gut Health

Your gut encompasses your digestive organs and all their resident microbes—and its health affects all the other systems in your body. Experience the physical and mental benefits of a healthy gut biome with this research-based guide. Find out how to care for your body, alleviate digestive distress, and soothe a wide variety of ailments, from heartburn and irritable bowel syndrome to depression and anxiety.

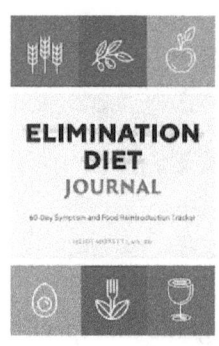

Elimination Diet Journal: 60-Day Symptom and Food Reintroduction Tracker

Your diet directly contributes to your health and sense of well-being, but some foods can cause inflammation, digestion issues, and aggravate autoimmune disorders. This journal will walk you through the elimination diet, giving you the tools and guidance to determine which foods are harming you and identify those that may help heal your gut.

Index

Symbols

2-Week Meal Plan, 222

5-Hydroxytryptophan, 74, 191

A

Air Fryer Salmon Rice Bowl, 261
Alcohol, 43, 95–96, 130, 156, 174, 208
Alpha Lipoic Acid, 75

Aromatase, 39, 140, 185, 272
Ashwagandha, 100, 121, 124–125, 165, 201, 203, 205

B

Berry-Yogurt, 268
Betaine, 69, 82, 201
Bioidentical Estrogen, 144
Bioidentical Progesterone, 142–143, 162–163,

Index

170, 173, 175, 198, 200
Birth Control, i–ii, v, 8, 11, 13, 21, 66, 71, 104, 110, 144, 151, 166, 175
Black Cohosh, 99, 122, 124, 194, 200–201, 203–206, 217, 270
Black Cumin Seed, 112–113, 170, 198, 207
Broccoli, 9, 38–41, 51, 53–54, 106, 110–111, 122, 145–146, 149, 169, 173, 188–190, 200, 222, 224, 226–227, 229, 233–234, 239–240, 246, 248–249, 256–257

Broccoli Salad, 224, 239–240
Burger Bowls, 224, 264
Butter Chicken, 225, 262
Buttery Sauteed Beets, 225, 240

C

Caffeine, 43, 76, 106
Calcitriol, 17, 25, 68, 82
Calcium, 51, 56, 58, 61, 122, 145, 150, 177, 183, 188–189, 191, 210, 276
Cannabis, 96, 106–109, 130, 148, 150, 163,

Index

195, 198, 201, 207, 215, 217
Carbohydrates, 22, 49–50, 66, 167, 221, 273, 275
Cholesterol, 23, 33–34, 44, 52, 101, 105, 174, 277
Chromium, 74, 86
Cinnamon, 113, 134–135, 161, 164, 170–171, 184, 245, 268–269
Cortisol, 17–20, 22–24, 27, 66, 91, 100–101, 112, 133, 193, 196, 198, 202–204, 216–217, 273, 277
Cortisol Steal, 19, 91, 273
Creamy Chicken with Mushrooms, 224, 257

D

Damiana, 120–121, 140, 174, 194, 198, 201, 214, 227
Dandelion Root, 102, 119, 146–147, 194
DHEA, 17–18, 27, 31, 46, 49, 147, 171, 190, 200, 205, 209–210, 270, 273, 277
Dietary Supplements, 32, 59, 70, 167, 180, 189, 280

Index

Dong Quai, 117, 122, 194, 201, 205
DUTCH Test, 18–19, 205

E

Eating Disorders, 151–154, 166
Endometriosis, 13, 27, 70, 72, 102, 105, 141, 151–152, 157–165, 173, 178–183, 196, 203, 273, 276
Energy, 19, 24, 26, 37, 50, 62, 106, 112, 119, 168, 193, 206, 221, 240, 275, 278
Estrogen, 17–18, 21–27, 29–30, 38–46, 53–54, 56–58, 63–68, 70, 73–74, 77, 79, 82, 84, 91, 99–100, 102, 104, 111, 113, 115, 119, 135, 142, 144–146, 148–149, 158, 160, 162, 167, 169, 171, 173–175, 190, 197, 200, 202–204, 272–274, 276–277

F

Fasting, 48, 112–113, 167–169, 172, 202, 275

Index

Fermented Foods, 42, 156, 193

Fermented Rice, 221, 223–224, 229, 244, 254, 256

Fermented Vegetables, 42, 193, 226, 242

Fibroids, 102, 171–175, 184–185, 196, 274

Fibromyalgia, 38, 274

Fluffy Egg Muffins, 226, 231

Folate, 37, 53, 71, 83–84, 164

G

Ginger, 110, 132–133, 146–147, 156, 162–163, 194, 201, 213, 228–229, 261–263

Ginkgo, 115–116, 122, 135–136, 170, 194, 201, 205–206, 213–214

Gluten, 21, 28, 50–51, 58, 62, 74, 154–156, 158–159, 169, 177–179, 222, 258, 264

Greek Salad, 229, 238

Gut Balance, 42

Index

H

Healing Foods, 32, 167
Healthy Chicken Nuggets, 228, 251
Healthy Fats, 24, 44–46, 48, 200, 221
Healthy Honey Lemonade/Limeade, 266
Heavy Flow, 6, 62, 147
Heavy Pain, 6
Heavy Period, 8, 10, 23, 34, 37, 60–62, 64–65, 98, 118, 141–142, 146–149, 151, 167, 172, 196, 274
High Protein, 268
Homemade Pesto, 260
Honey-Garlic Shrimp and Broccoli, 226, 256
Hormone Detoxifiers, 38, 42
Hormone Testing, 18
Hormones, i–ii, 8, 11–20, 22–30, 32–34, 36–38, 42–44, 47–48, 50–51, 55, 57, 63–64, 66–74, 77, 81, 85, 91, 102–103, 106, 109, 112–114, 142–145, 150, 155, 159–160, 169–170, 172, 174–175, 177, 188, 190, 193, 196–198, 200, 205, 220, 248,

Index

256–257, 267–268, 273–274, 276–277
Hot Flashes, 99, 102–103, 109, 112, 115–117, 122, 124, 127, 131–132, 136, 194, 201–205, 207, 217, 277

I

Indoles, 38, 40–41
Inflammation, 18–19, 37, 66, 69, 73–74, 83, 91, 101–102, 110–112, 114, 119, 126, 150, 157–161, 163, 167–170, 172–174, 178, 184–185, 192, 196, 202–204, 207–208, 241, 272, 275–277, 281
Inositol, 75–76, 87–88, 129, 170
Insulin, 17, 19–22, 24–25, 29, 37–38, 47–49, 57, 63, 67–68, 70, 73–76, 82–83, 87–88, 112–113, 119, 126, 134, 166–168, 170–173, 184–185, 190, 196, 202, 210, 216, 273, 275–276
Insulin Resistance, 22, 25, 29, 57, 70,

Index

73–76, 87–88, 113, 126, 134, 166–168, 171, 196, 202, 216, 275

Iodine, 21, 76–78, 88, 156

Iron, 21, 34, 36–37, 60–63, 65, 78, 146–147, 149, 155, 174, 192, 198–200, 211, 234, 246, 255

Irregular Periods, 34, 49, 102, 141, 151–152, 155, 166, 171

L

L-Tyrosine, 74, 86, 191–192, 201

Lemony Dressing, 223–224, 226, 228, 236

Licorice Root, 122, 156, 161, 204–205, 224

Liver, 34–38, 44–45, 52, 63–65, 69, 71, 78, 101–102, 119, 122, 139, 145–147, 158, 161, 173, 177, 189–190, 192, 198–200, 222–223, 228, 255–256, 263–265

Liver, Vodka, and Onions, 228, 255

Index

M

Maca, 106, 122, 205–206
Meal Balance, 221
Meatballs with Nourishing Beef Liver, 223, 263
Memory, 75, 100–101, 111, 115–116, 192, 201, 206
Menopause, 25, 27, 46, 75, 82, 99–100, 102–103, 112, 115–116, 122–124, 128–129, 131–132, 134, 137, 143, 147, 149, 175, 187, 190, 198, 201–203, 205–207, 209, 215–217, 274
Menstrual Migraines, 142, 207–208
Menstrual Pain, 44–45, 52, 55, 75, 107, 113, 117, 148–150
Milk Thistle, 9, 101–102, 122, 145–146, 165, 170, 173, 203, 205–206
Mittelschmerz, 9, 144–145, 275
Motherwort, 117–118, 137–138, 149, 155, 164, 199, 201, 206
Mushrooms, 75, 87, 206, 224, 232–234, 246, 257–258, 272

Index

N

Natural Hormone Detoxifiers, 38
Natural Medicine, ii–iii, 9–10, 12, 45, 97, 127, 202, 278
Nettles, 116, 156, 201, 205

O

Omega 3, 44–45, 164, 256
Organ Meats, 34, 62, 64–65, 73, 75, 155, 163, 189–190, 198–200, 203
Ovary Pain, 9

P

Passion Flower, 118, 122, 165, 194, 201, 206
PCOS, 26, 37, 39, 47, 49, 65–66, 68, 70, 74–76, 87–88, 98, 101–102, 105, 112–113, 115, 122, 142–143, 151–152, 166–171, 174, 183, 196
Perfect Sauteed Broccoli, 248
Perimenopause, 25, 100, 102, 105, 121–122, 124, 142–143, 151, 190, 195–201, 215
Period Problems, 24, 27, 32–33

Index

Pesto Salmon with Tomatoes, 258
Phytoestrogens, 165, 183, 276
Pine Bark, 105–106, 129, 150, 162, 181, 201, 205, 208, 218
PMS, 91, 99, 102–104, 109, 115, 117–118, 121–122, 131, 175, 187–189, 191–195, 198, 206, 210, 212
Polycystic Ovarian Syndrome, 13, 22, 24, 101, 141, 166, 173, 276
Premenstrual Syndrome, 16, 58, 73, 97, 126, 131, 136, 142, 187, 209–214
Probiotics, 42, 154, 160, 193, 276
Progesterone, 17–18, 21–27, 29–30, 37, 47, 54, 56, 64, 67, 70–71, 80, 86, 91, 98–99, 114, 119, 121, 135, 142–143, 147, 149, 158, 162–163, 167, 170–171, 173, 175–177, 182, 190, 196, 198–200, 203, 208, 273–275, 277
Protein, 21, 37, 43, 47–49, 51, 56–57, 80, 154–156, 200–201, 221, 256,

Index

268–269, 272, 275, 278

Q

Quercetin, 69–70, 83, 161, 164, 170, 174, 180

R

Red Raspberry Leaf, 104, 121, 147, 163–164, 225–229
Roasted Vegetables, 228, 246

S

Saffron, 91, 98, 122–123, 194, 198, 201, 206, 213
Sage, 96, 111–112, 122, 133, 174, 179, 201, 205–206, 228, 246, 250
Salsa Poached Eggs, 224, 234
Sauerkraut Recipe, 241
Sauteed Potatoes, 229, 231
Savory Slow-Cooker Pepper Steak, 253
Selenium, 21, 37, 71
Sexual Function, 24, 29, 100,

Index

105, 109, 120, 144, 201, 205, 209
Spicy Sweet Potato Hash Browns, 245
St. John's Wort, 109–110, 118, 131–132, 194, 201
Super Quick Sausage and Vegetables, 254
Sweet Potato Fries Air Fryer Style, 247

T

Testosterone, 17–19, 21, 24, 27, 30, 37–39, 49, 68, 76–77, 91, 104–105, 167–168, 171, 190, 272–273, 277
Thiamine, 73, 75, 85, 150, 155
Thyroid Hormone,, 21
Toxins, 35, 40, 69, 119, 190, 274
Tribulus, 104–105, 121, 128–129, 147, 170, 205
Tulsi, 101, 125, 170, 206, 223–227
Tuna Salad on Greens, 226, 237
Turmeric, 9, 102–103, 122, 145–147, 156, 160, 162, 164, 170, 173, 194, 198, 201, 206–207,

Index

262, 270

U

Uterine Fibroids, 171–172, 175, 184–185

V

Valerian Root, 103, 126–127, 194, 201, 205
Versatile Chicken Vegetable Soup, 250
Versatile Egg Pie Recipe, 233
Vitamin A, 37, 45, 53, 64–65, 78–79, 147, 149, 163, 189, 192, 200
Vitamin B1, 73, 75, 85
Vitamin B6, 37, 53, 71–72, 83, 122, 163, 189, 191, 200–201, 210
Vitamin B12, 36–37, 65, 71, 275
Vitamin C, 61, 66–67, 71, 78–81, 147, 150, 163, 189, 193
Vitamin D, 21, 25, 30, 58, 65, 67–68, 77, 81–82, 169, 172, 179, 182, 184, 189, 191, 200, 210–211
Vitamin E, 45, 53, 65, 72, 84–85, 147, 150, 163,

Index

189, 192, 211, 217

Vitex, 97–98, 109, 121–123, 131, 146–147, 149, 163, 170–171, 175, 182, 194, 198, 201, 208, 213, 270

161, 181, 190, 192, 211, 276

W

Wholesome Chocolates, 267

Z

Zinc, 21, 37, 51, 71–72, 84, 122, 150,

Index

Symbols

2-Week Meal Plan, 222

5-Hydroxytryptophan, 74, 191

A

Air Fryer Salmon Rice Bowl, 261
Alcohol, 43, 95–96, 130, 156, 174, 208
Alpha Lipoic Acid, 75
Aromatase, 39, 140, 185, 272
Ashwagandha, 100, 121, 124–125, 165, 201, 203, 205

B

Berry-Yogurt, 268
Betaine, 69, 82, 201
Bioidentical Estrogen, 144
Bioidentical Progesterone, 142–143, 162–163,

Index

170, 173, 175, 198, 200
Birth Control, i–ii, v, 8, 11, 13, 21, 66, 71, 104, 110, 144, 151, 166, 175
Black Cohosh, 99, 122, 124, 194, 200–201, 203–206, 217, 270
Black Cumin Seed, 112–113, 170, 198, 207
Broccoli, 9, 38–41, 51, 53–54, 106, 110–111, 122, 145–146, 149, 169, 173, 188–190, 200, 222, 224, 226–227, 229, 233–234, 239–240, 246, 248–249, 256–257

Broccoli Salad, 224, 239–240
Burger Bowls, 224, 264
Butter Chicken, 225, 262
Buttery Sauteed Beets, 225, 240

C

Caffeine, 43, 76, 106
Calcitriol, 17, 25, 68, 82
Calcium, 51, 56, 58, 61, 122, 145, 150, 177, 183, 188–189, 191, 210, 276
Cannabis, 96, 106–109, 130, 148, 150, 163,

Index

195, 198, 201, 207, 215, 217

Carbohydrates, 22, 49–50, 66, 167, 221, 273, 275

Cholesterol, 23, 33–34, 44, 52, 101, 105, 174, 277

Chromium, 74, 86

Cinnamon, 113, 134–135, 161, 164, 170–171, 184, 245, 268–269

Cortisol, 17–20, 22–24, 27, 66, 91, 100–101, 112, 133, 193, 196, 198, 202–204, 216–217, 273, 277

Cortisol Steal, 19, 91, 273

Creamy Chicken with Mushrooms, 224, 257

D

Damiana, 120–121, 140, 174, 194, 198, 201, 214, 227

Dandelion Root, 102, 119, 146–147, 194

DHEA, 17–18, 27, 31, 46, 49, 147, 171, 190, 200, 205, 209–210, 270, 273, 277

Dietary Supplements, 32, 59, 70, 167, 180, 189, 280

Index

Dong Quai, 117, 122, 194, 201, 205
DUTCH Test, 18–19, 205

E

Eating Disorders, 151–154, 166
Endometriosis, 13, 27, 70, 72, 102, 105, 141, 151–152, 157–165, 173, 178–183, 196, 203, 273, 276
Energy, 19, 24, 26, 37, 50, 62, 106, 112, 119, 168, 193, 206, 221, 240, 275, 278
Estrogen, 17–18, 21–27, 29–30, 38–46, 53–54, 56–58, 63–68, 70, 73–74, 77, 79, 82, 84, 91, 99–100, 102, 104, 111, 113, 115, 119, 135, 142, 144–146, 148–149, 158, 160, 162, 167, 169, 171, 173–175, 190, 197, 200, 202–204, 272–274, 276–277

F

Fasting, 48, 112–113, 167–169, 172, 202, 275

Index

Fermented Foods, 42, 156, 193
Fermented Rice, 221, 223–224, 229, 244, 254, 256
Fermented Vegetables, 42, 193, 226, 242
Fibroids, 102, 171–175, 184–185, 196, 274
Fibromyalgia, 38, 274
Fluffy Egg Muffins, 226, 231
Folate, 37, 53, 71, 83–84, 164

G

Ginger, 110, 132–133, 146–147, 156, 162–163, 194, 201, 213, 228–229, 261–263
Ginkgo, 115–116, 122, 135–136, 170, 194, 201, 205–206, 213–214
Gluten, 21, 28, 50–51, 58, 62, 74, 154–156, 158–159, 169, 177–179, 222, 258, 264
Greek Salad, 229, 238
Gut Balance, 42

Index

H

Healing Foods, 32, 167
Healthy Chicken Nuggets, 228, 251
Healthy Fats, 24, 44–46, 48, 200, 221
Healthy Honey Lemonade/Limeade, 266
Heavy Flow, 6, 62, 147
Heavy Pain, 6
Heavy Period, 8, 10, 23, 34, 37, 60–62, 64–65, 98, 118, 141–142, 146–149, 151, 167, 172, 196, 274
High Protein, 268
Homemade Pesto, 260
Honey-Garlic Shrimp and Broccoli, 226, 256
Hormone Detoxifiers, 38, 42
Hormone Testing, 18
Hormones, i–ii, 8, 11–20, 22–30, 32–34, 36–38, 42–44, 47–48, 50–51, 55, 57, 63–64, 66–74, 77, 81, 85, 91, 102–103, 106, 109, 112–114, 142–145, 150, 155, 159–160, 169–170, 172, 174–175, 177, 188, 190, 193, 196–198, 200, 205, 220, 248,

Index

256–257, 267–268, 273–274, 276–277
Hot Flashes, 99, 102–103, 109, 112, 115–117, 122, 124, 127, 131–132, 136, 194, 201–205, 207, 217, 277

I

Indoles, 38, 40–41
Inflammation, 18–19, 37, 66, 69, 73–74, 83, 91, 101–102, 110–112, 114, 119, 126, 150, 157–161, 163, 167–170, 172–174, 178, 184–185, 192, 196, 202–204, 207–208, 241, 272, 275–277, 281
Inositol, 75–76, 87–88, 129, 170
Insulin, 17, 19–22, 24–25, 29, 37–38, 47–49, 57, 63, 67–68, 70, 73–76, 82–83, 87–88, 112–113, 119, 126, 134, 166–168, 170–173, 184–185, 190, 196, 202, 210, 216, 273, 275–276
Insulin Resistance, 22, 25, 29, 57, 70,

Index

73–76, 87–88, 113, 126, 134, 166–168, 171, 196, 202, 216, 275

Iodine, 21, 76–78, 88, 156

Iron, 21, 34, 36–37, 60–63, 65, 78, 146–147, 149, 155, 174, 192, 198–200, 211, 234, 246, 255

Irregular Periods, 34, 49, 102, 141, 151–152, 155, 166, 171

Lemony Dressing, 223–224, 226, 228, 236

Licorice Root, 122, 156, 161, 204–205, 224

Liver, 34–38, 44–45, 52, 63–65, 69, 71, 78, 101–102, 119, 122, 139, 145–147, 158, 161, 173, 177, 189–190, 192, 198–200, 222–223, 228, 255–256, 263–265

Liver, Vodka, and Onions, 228, 255

L

L-Tyrosine, 74, 86, 191–192, 201

Index

M

Maca, 106, 122, 205–206
Meal Balance, 221
Meatballs with Nourishing Beef Liver, 223, 263
Memory, 75, 100–101, 111, 115–116, 192, 201, 206
Menopause, 25, 27, 46, 75, 82, 99–100, 102–103, 112, 115–116, 122–124, 128–129, 131–132, 134, 137, 143, 147, 149, 175, 187, 190, 198, 201–203, 205–207, 209, 215–217, 274
Menstrual Migraines, 142, 207–208
Menstrual Pain, 44–45, 52, 55, 75, 107, 113, 117, 148–150
Milk Thistle, 9, 101–102, 122, 145–146, 165, 170, 173, 203, 205–206
Mittelschmerz, 9, 144–145, 275
Motherwort, 117–118, 137–138, 149, 155, 164, 199, 201, 206
Mushrooms, 75, 87, 206, 224, 232–234, 246, 257–258, 272

Index

N

Natural Hormone Detoxifiers, 38
Natural Medicine, ii–iii, 9–10, 12, 45, 97, 127, 202, 278
Nettles, 116, 156, 201, 205

O

Omega 3, 44–45, 164, 256
Organ Meats, 34, 62, 64–65, 73, 75, 155, 163, 189–190, 198–200, 203
Ovary Pain, 9

P

Passion Flower, 118, 122, 165, 194, 201, 206
PCOS, 26, 37, 39, 47, 49, 65–66, 68, 70, 74–76, 87–88, 98, 101–102, 105, 112–113, 115, 122, 142–143, 151–152, 166–171, 174, 183, 196
Perfect Sauteed Broccoli, 248
Perimenopause, 25, 100, 102, 105, 121–122, 124, 142–143, 151, 190, 195–201, 215
Period Problems, 24, 27, 32–33

Index

Pesto Salmon with Tomatoes, 258
Phytoestrogens, 165, 183, 276
Pine Bark, 105–106, 129, 150, 162, 181, 201, 205, 208, 218
PMS, 91, 99, 102–104, 109, 115, 117–118, 121–122, 131, 175, 187–189, 191–195, 198, 206, 210, 212
Polycystic Ovarian Syndrome, 13, 22, 24, 101, 141, 166, 173, 276
Premenstrual Syndrome, 16, 58, 73, 97, 126, 131, 136, 142, 187, 209–214
Probiotics, 42, 154, 160, 193, 276
Progesterone, 17–18, 21–27, 29–30, 37, 47, 54, 56, 64, 67, 70–71, 80, 86, 91, 98–99, 114, 119, 121, 135, 142–143, 147, 149, 158, 162–163, 167, 170–171, 173, 175–177, 182, 190, 196, 198–200, 203, 208, 273–275, 277
Protein, 21, 37, 43, 47–49, 51, 56–57, 80, 154–156, 200–201, 221, 256,

Index

268–269, 272, 275, 278

Q

Quercetin, 69–70, 83, 161, 164, 170, 174, 180

R

Red Raspberry Leaf, 104, 121, 147, 163–164, 225–229

Roasted Vegetables, 228, 246

S

Saffron, 91, 98, 122–123, 194, 198, 201, 206, 213

Sage, 96, 111–112, 122, 133, 174, 179, 201, 205–206, 228, 246, 250

Salsa Poached Eggs, 224, 234

Sauerkraut Recipe, 241

Sauteed Potatoes, 229, 231

Savory Slow-Cooker Pepper Steak, 253

Selenium, 21, 37, 71

Sexual Function, 24, 29, 100,

Index

105, 109, 120, 144, 201, 205, 209
Spicy Sweet Potato Hash Browns, 245
St. John's Wort, 109–110, 118, 131–132, 194, 201
Super Quick Sausage and Vegetables, 254
Sweet Potato Fries Air Fryer Style, 247

T

Testosterone, 17–19, 21, 24, 27, 30, 37–39, 49, 68, 76–77, 91, 104–105, 167–168, 171, 190, 272–273, 277
Thiamine, 73, 75, 85, 150, 155
Thyroid Hormone,, 21
Toxins, 35, 40, 69, 119, 190, 274
Tribulus, 104–105, 121, 128–129, 147, 170, 205
Tulsi, 101, 125, 170, 206, 223–227
Tuna Salad on Greens, 226, 237
Turmeric, 9, 102–103, 122, 145–147, 156, 160, 162, 164, 170, 173, 194, 198, 201, 206–207,

Index

262, 270

U

Uterine Fibroids, 171–172, 175, 184–185

V

Valerian Root, 103, 126–127, 194, 201, 205
Versatile Chicken Vegetable Soup, 250
Versatile Egg Pie Recipe, 233
Vitamin A, 37, 45, 53, 64–65, 78–79, 147, 149, 163, 189, 192, 200
Vitamin B1, 73, 75, 85
Vitamin B6, 37, 53, 71–72, 83, 122, 163, 189, 191, 200–201, 210
Vitamin B12, 36–37, 65, 71, 275
Vitamin C, 61, 66–67, 71, 78–81, 147, 150, 163, 189, 193
Vitamin D, 21, 25, 30, 58, 65, 67–68, 77, 81–82, 169, 172, 179, 182, 184, 189, 191, 200, 210–211
Vitamin E, 45, 53, 65, 72, 84–85, 147, 150, 163,

Index

189, 192, 211, 217
Vitex, 97–98, 109, 121–123, 131, 146–147, 149, 163, 170–171, 175, 182, 194, 198, 201, 208, 213, 270

161, 181, 190, 192, 211, 276

W

Wholesome Chocolates, 267

Z

Zinc, 21, 37, 51, 71–72, 84, 122, 150,

www.ingramcontent.com/pod-product-compliance
Lightning Source LLC
Chambersburg PA
CBHW060451030426
42337CB00015B/1554